Health Care in Transition

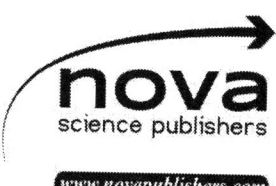

Health Care in Transition

**Mobile Health: Advances in Research
and Applications – Volume II**
Gaurav Gupta, PhD, Varun Jaiswal, PhD,
Manju Khari, PhD, Nagesh Kumar, PhD (Editors)
2022 ISBN: 978-1-68507-988-8 (Hardcover)
2022 ISBN: 979-8-88697-247-4 (eBook)

**Novel Perspectives in Economics of Personalized
Medicine and Healthcare Systems**
Marinko Škare, PhD, Romina Pržiklas Družeta, PhD,
Sandra Kraljević Pavelić, PhD (Editors)
2021 ISBN: 978-1-68507-390-9 (Hardcover)
2021 ISBN: 978-1-68507-393-0 (eBook)

**Driving Hospitals Towards Performance:
Practical Managerial Guidance to Reach
the "Perfect Symphony"**
Irene Gabutti, PhD
2021 ISBN: 978-1-68507-225-4 (Softcover)
2021 ISBN: 978-1-68507-382-4 (eBook)

**Blockchain and Health: Transformation
of Care and Impact of Digitalization**
Jan Veuger, PhD (Editor)
2021 ISBN: 978-1-68507-232-2 (Hardcover)
2021 ISBN: 978-1-68507-260-5 (eBook)

Environmental Health in Malaysia
Hisham Atan Edinur, PhD,
Mohd Tajuddin Abdullah, PhD,
Sabreena Safuan, PhD (Editors)
2021 ISBN: 978-1-68507-114-1 (Hardcover)
2021 ISBN: 978-1-68507-136-3 (eBook)

More information about this series can be found at
https://novapublishers.com/product-category/series/health-care-in-transition/.

Behrouz Ehsani-Moghaddam

Handbook of Data Analysis of Electronic Health Records (EHR) Using SAS® Software

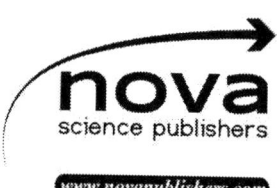

www.novapublishers.com

Copyright © 2023 by Nova Science Publishers, Inc.
DOI: 10.52305/BXKA2663.

All rights reserved. No part of this book may be reproduced, stored in a retrieval system or transmitted in any form or by any means: electronic, electrostatic, magnetic, tape, mechanical photocopying, recording or otherwise without the written permission of the Publisher.

We have partnered with Copyright Clearance Center to make it easy for you to obtain permissions to reuse content from this publication. Simply navigate to this publication's page on Nova's website and locate the "Get Permission" button below the title description. This button is linked directly to the title's permission page on copyright.com. Alternatively, you can visit copyright.com and search by title, ISBN, or ISSN.

For further questions about using the service on copyright.com, please contact:
Copyright Clearance Center
Phone: +1-(978) 750-8400   Fax: +1-(978) 750-4470   E-mail: info@copyright.com.

NOTICE TO THE READER

The Publisher has taken reasonable care in the preparation of this book, but makes no expressed or implied warranty of any kind and assumes no responsibility for any errors or omissions. No liability is assumed for incidental or consequential damages in connection with or arising out of information contained in this book. The Publisher shall not be liable for any special, consequential, or exemplary damages resulting, in whole or in part, from the readers' use of, or reliance upon, this material. Any parts of this book based on government reports are so indicated and copyright is claimed for those parts to the extent applicable to compilations of such works.

Independent verification should be sought for any data, advice or recommendations contained in this book. In addition, no responsibility is assumed by the Publisher for any injury and/or damage to persons or property arising from any methods, products, instructions, ideas or otherwise contained in this publication.

This publication is designed to provide accurate and authoritative information with regard to the subject matter covered herein. It is sold with the clear understanding that the Publisher is not engaged in rendering legal or any other professional services. If legal or any other expert assistance is required, the services of a competent person should be sought. FROM A DECLARATION OF PARTICIPANTS JOINTLY ADOPTED BY A COMMITTEE OF THE AMERICAN BAR ASSOCIATION AND A COMMITTEE OF PUBLISHERS.

Additional color graphics may be available in the e-book version of this book.

Library of Congress Cataloging-in-Publication Data

ISBN: 979-8-88697-372-3

Published by Nova Science Publishers, Inc. † New York

*To my mom, Zahra,
and to my family, Forough and Roxana*

Contents

Preface ix

Part I: Basic Information about EHR Data and Data Manipulation 1

Chapter 1   EHR Observations 3

Chapter 2   Data Transfer from Database Management Systems to SAS 15

Chapter 3   Creating Temporary and Permanent Data Sets 27

Chapter 4   Retrieving Patient Information 43

Part II: Analysis of Longitudinal EHR Data 67

Chapter 5   Data Extraction from Text and Analysis: Adverse Events Following Immunization 69

Chapter 6   Prevalence Estimation for Acute Diseases (A Cross-Sectional Cohort Study) 85

Chapter 7   Prevalence Estimation for Chronic Diseases 103

Chapter 8   Disease Case Validation 119

Chapter 9   Multiple Logistic Regression 131

Chapter 10   Machine Learning for Medical Diagnoses 141

Index 165

About the Author 169

Preface

Over the past decade, as medical digital records replaced paper files across the world, the size and complexity of records also increased. In Electronic Medical Record (EMR) and Electronic Health Record (EHR), patient information such as demographic, medication, health problem and ICD codes are distributed across several datasets such as Patient, Medication, Billing, Encounter Diagnosis, Health Condition, Vaccination, Referral, Lab results, etc. These data are longitudinal records that are stored in a database that follows current and new patients at different points in time. Since EHR data come from multiple different vendors and open-source products, they can be messy, inconsistent, and often need to be harmonized and reformatted properly before they can provide real-world perceptions about patients using statistical techniques. To achieve reliable and useful information from these non-standard data and to perform basic statistical analysis one needs to know basic SAS programming for this type of data. Unfortunately, very few researchers and even statisticians have hands-on experience with both EHR data and SAS program.

  This book is a hands-on tutorial for those SAS users with little or no experience with EHR database and little experience with the programming language. The book covers all necessary and practical steps that healthcare researchers or practitioners need to know in order to analyze electronic big data, such as importation of unstructured (texts) or structured patient information (ICD codes, diseases diagnosis, demographic variables, etc.) from Microsoft SQL server or other data management servers into SAS software, data quality evaluation such as cleaning of data including removing duplicate records, detecting and modifying mismatched observations, identifying outliers and incorrect data and dropping unnecessary variables, then using merging or appending techniques to merge encounter records of patients with their demographic available records and creating new variables. The book also covers statistical analysis to estimate prevalence of diseases including prevalence estimation of chronic and non-chronic diseases, sex-age standardization, creating and selecting statistical models, risk and odds ratio estimation, regression, data simulation, model performance evaluation, sensitivity analysis (sensitivity, specificity, positive predictive value, accuracy, Kappa, etc.), disease case validation and machine learning.

Part I: Basic Information about EHR Data and Data Manipulation

Chapter 1

EHR Observations

Abstract

The use of digital health records has been accelerating over the years as healthcare organizations are trying to provide greater quality care to patients. While there are some differences between an Electronic Medical Record (EMR) and an Electronic Health Record (EHR), perhaps the major difference between these two systems is the volume and completeness of the information that they collect. EMR is held by individual and independent health providers that often cover an incomplete medical record that may contain only a portion of information from a single clinic or provider about a person over a lifetime. The EMR information from one provider is not supposed to be shared with another provider. It is more restricted to a specific location. In EHR, a person's information is gathered from multiple providers; therefore, heath practitioners can get access to more comprehensive patient health records. Unlike EMR, there is no restriction of location in EHR system as they have been designed to share patient's information between different healthcare providers. Basically, an EHR is an EMR with its ability to integrate with other providers' systems.

Both EMR and EHR systems help healthcare providers and decision makers to keep patient information safe, organized, up-to-date, accurate, and suitable for processing by statistical software, resulting an overall improvement in the quality of care and patient outcomes. Many healthcare experts use EHR and EMR interchangeably. EHR is used in this book for simplicity as all techniques that are shown and discussed can be applied to both systems. After completing this chapter, you will know:

- EHR definition and its structure
- Data quality including data dimensions and security
- Different types of variables
- Record Linkage and its usage

1.1. EHR Definition

This book utilizes the following EHR definition that is suggested by the Health Information Management Systems Society's (HIMSS):

> The Electronic Health Record (EHR) is a longitudinal electronic record of patient health information generated by one or more encounters in any care delivery setting. Included in this information are patient demographics, progress notes, problems, medications, vital signs, past medical history, immunizations, laboratory data and radiology reports. The EHR automates and streamlines the clinician's workflow. The EHR has the ability to generate a complete record of a clinical patient encounter - as well as supporting other care-related activities directly or indirectly via interface - including evidence-based decision support, quality management, and outcomes reporting.

1.2. Structure of EHR Data

For each service (encounter) that a patient receives from a healthcare provider, an electronic health record is created. The service can be administrative, clinical, pharmacy, vaccination, radiology, laboratory, etc. The captured records are stored in a silo system by different vendors. Each vendor has its own standard of vocabulary variation, patient identification (ID) number, etc. Every time a new record is available electronically, it is added to the old records.

In a process of incorporation, the system resolves many terminology variations. For example, if patients are diagnosed with "A disorder characterized by difficulty in falling asleep and/or remaining asleep" or "waking up too early" or "the patient has symptoms of insomnia," these three indications are incorporated into a single term as "insomnia." Since patient information can be entered in different methods such as in a structured form, free texts, images, and so on, therefore, there must be a structured vocabulary system that can resolve the vocabulary variations. In addition to the structured vocabulary system, the record must be entered in such a way that the system can recognize the correct terms and place them in the context. The systems that use concepts or terminologies not appropriately selected for the field will not produce useful information. That is why sometimes a huge portion of an EHR is useless, which causes poor data quality.

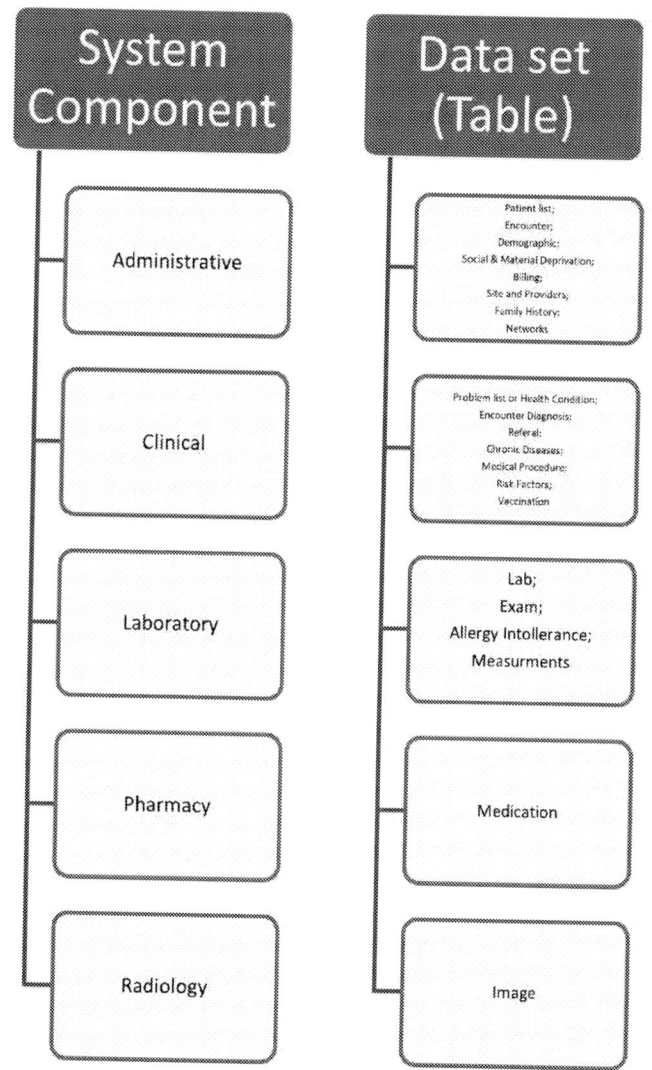

Figure 1.1. The structure of a typical EHR data quality and security.

EHRs are designed to integrate data from the large supplementary services, such as administration, laboratory, pharmacy, vaccination, and referral. In every life cycle of the EHR database, records of patients are updated with new information which is collected at the most recent encounters and entered into several data sets (tables), such as billing, encounter diagnosis, problem list (health condition), vaccination and so on. Figure 1.1 illustrates the structure of a typical EHR. The resulting data sets are the product of integration of medical and socioeconomic data from several system components (supplementary services). The number of system components and data sets may increase or decrease in accordance with the available resources and necessities.

1.3. The Structure of a Typical EHR Data Quality and Security

The value of healthcare data depends deeply on data properties such as accuracy and precision, completeness and comprehensiveness, consistency, timeliness, uniqueness, data cleaning and coherence. These data properties can outline the concept of data quality. Data quality can also be defined within the context of an intended data user's needs. These data users can be graduate students, academic researchers, healthcare providers, health agencies, health system planners, decision makers and industry partners. In general, data quality is the degree to which a given dataset meets a user's requirements. To extract reliable and beneficial information from a large quantity of data and to make more effective and informed decisions, data should be as clean and free of errors as possible (Ehsani-Moghaddam et al., 2019). The quality of healthcare data is important, not only from patient care perspective, but also for monitoring the performance of the health services.

Poor data quality has some negative consequences. For healthcare providers and decision support systems, incorrect decisions made by poor quality of data can mean the difference between life and death. The various ways of assessing the quality of data depend upon the dimensionality of the data such as number of observations, available independent and dependent variables and the requirements of the intended study (Weiskopf et al., 2017).

1.3.1. EHR Data Quality

As a good practice, data managers, analysts, and EHR users should investigate and review data quality in a regular basis or prior to utilize data for research projects as EHR data are created primarily for the benefit of practitioners such as physicians and not for research or analytics. Therefore,

EHR data often require extensive cleaning and preparation before being used for analysis. In this section, you will be introduced to some of the most important dimensions of data quality in EHR.

1.3.1.1. Accuracy and Precision

Accuracy refers to the rightness of the information and how close quantities are to the "true" value. Precision refers to how close quantities are to each other. Although accuracy and precision are not the same, however, accuracy sometimes is measured by precision parameters such as sensitivity and specificity. In data, estimation of accuracy of independent variables is challenging and sometimes even impossible. For dependent variables such as incidence of diseases with binary outcomes, the accuracy of data can be estimated and validated from a confusion matrix using the following formula:

Accuracy = (True Positive + True Negative) / (True Positive + True Negative + False Positive + False Negative)

1.3.1.2. Coherence

Coherence over time reflects the degree to which the data are logically connected and mutually consistent (OECD, 2017). Incoherence shows disruptions in a series resulting from changes in perceptions, classifications, and methodology. The consistency of EHR database should be evaluated on a regular basis by several methods. First, by simple comparisons between the new version and previous version, for some data attributes such as the size, number of observations and number of variables for different tables (Billing, Vaccination, etc.). Prevalence estimation of some random diseases over years can be a very good indication of possible fluctuation in data flow. By estimation of prevalence, the coherence is monitored over several years to make sure that the incidence/prevalence of the disease for each data life cycle is as expected statistically. The consistency of variable characteristics over time is also examined. For example, Site-ID or Patient-ID should be unique and consistence over time for the same site or for the same patient and have the same attributes such as the same length, size, and label and either character or numeric, but not both.

1.3.1.3. Completeness and Comprehensiveness

Completeness is the percentage of non-missing data available for a specific requirement. A measure of data completeness is the percentage of missing data. Comprehensiveness means that all required data items for a particular use must be included and available to users (AHIMA, 2012) and that the record is complete and covers all relevant information. It can also be referred to as inclusiveness or being able to represent the entire population. The predictive ability of any model including machine learning algorithms depends heavily on the number of independent variables and can be increased by employing data sets that contain higher completeness and comprehensive relevant information. Therefore, greater completeness and comprehensiveness, better data quality.

1.3.1.4. Consistency
Consistency is the measure of the absence of variations between the data items representing the same objects across applications and systems. Data consistency can refer to individual observations or units of measurements. For example, the unit for patient height should be the same across different records, either meter or feet, but not both.

1.3.1.5. Data Cleaning
EHR data are created primarily for the benefit of practitioners such as physicians and not researchers or analysts. This is why we often see poorly structured data in EHR such as having free text in fields where a data set is defined for analysis. Since EHR data come from multiple vendors and open-source products, they can be messy and inconsistent and need to be harmonized and reformatted properly before you can perform analysis and provide real-world insights about patients. Therefore, in most cases, prior to analysis data cleaning should be carried out. The process of data cleaning may include but not limited to identifying the types of errors and unreliable information causing poor data quality and correcting or removing such inconsistencies, then detecting and removing unwanted or unnecessary information, variables, and columns.

1.3.1.6. Randomness
Data randomness refers to absence of patterns in observations. An EHR data that represents the entire population does not show any significant pattern. In the absence of randomness in EHR, selection bias may happen, which means some patients are more likely to be in the sample than others. When selection bias happens, you can still make inferences about the patients in the sample, but not about the entire population.

5. *Limiting use, disclosure, and retention of personal health information.* When organizations identify the purposes for which they collect PHI and seek the appropriate consent for these purposes, it is vital that they then only use, disclose, and retain information for these purposes.
6. *Accuracy of personal health information.* The requirement for accuracy as a fair information practice has particular relevance for the delivery of healthcare to patients/persons, who share with organizations a commitment to accuracy in order to ensure efficient and effective delivery of healthcare.
7. *Safeguards for the protection of personal health information.* The EHR, organizations connecting to the EHR and organizations hosting components of the EHR must protect PHI, through the application of appropriate security safeguards, against loss or theft, as well as unauthorized access, disclosure, copying, use, or modification.
8. *Openness about practices concerning the management of personal health information.* Organizations connecting to the EHR or hosting components of the EHR must make readily available to the public specific information about their policies and practices relating to the management of PHI. At minimum, they should make available information such as the name or title, and the address, of the person who is accountable for the organization's policies, the means by which patients/persons can gain access to EHR, a description of the personal information held by the organization, a general description of the administrative, technical and physical safeguards and practices the organization maintains for PHI and what PHI is made available to related organizations.
9. *Individual access to personal health information.* Patients have a legal right of access to their own health information, subject to limited exceptions in specified circumstances.
10. *Challenging compliance.* The right of any patient/person to lodge a privacy complaint is a core fair information practice. Organizations connecting to or hosting components of the EHR must easily be accessible and simple-to-use procedures in place to receive and respond to complaints or inquiries about their policies and practices relating to the handling of PHI.

1.4. Types of Variables

EHR captures different types of variables, such as patient identifiers (patient-ID, date of birth, postal code), demographics (age, gender, ethnicity, etc.), diagnoses, problem lists, medications, procedure (surgery), laboratory data (often as the Logical Observation Identifiers Names and Codes or LOINC), vital measurements (e.g., height, weight, body mass index, blood pressure), risk factors (e.g., smoking status, alcohol consumption), socio-economic status (housing condition, social and material deprivation, employment status) and dates (date of onset for disease or medication, encounter date, service date, etc.). Diagnosis includes symptoms of a disease, disease name and the International Classification of Diseases (ICD) and sometimes unstructured data (e.g., clinical notes) that can be further processed to extract useful data.

In general, variables or so-called features in machine learning studies can be divided into independent and dependent variables. The independent variable is the variable that influences the outcome. A dependent variable is the result or outcome of the independent variable. Sometimes an independent variable is called predictor, explanatory, or exposure variable and a dependent variable is called an outcome or response variable. For example, in a study, you want to investigate the effect of different anticoagulants on the prevalence of heart stroke. Anticoagulant medication is considered as an independent variable or feature and the prevalence of stroke is called dependent variable.

In terms of characteristics, variables can be defined as categorical (discrete or qualitative) and continuous variables. Categorical variables can be further categorized as either nominal, ordinal or dichotomous. Nominal variables are variables that have two or more categories without a natural order or ranking. For example, blood type is a nominal variable. Dichotomous variables are categorical variables that have only two levels. For example, patient's gender can be categorized as either male or female. Ordinal variables are like nominal variables in that they can be categorized in two or more levels, but unlike nominal variables the categories can also be ordered or ranked. For example, Body Mass Index (BMI) in adult patients can be categorized as underweight, normal, overweight, and obese.

Every EHR database should be accompanied by a data dictionary. The purpose of the data dictionary is making users to become familiar with the type of data that is collected within the database including variables formats, structure, percentage of missing data, and some other important information. Table 1.1 shows a small portion of a data dictionary for an EHR database.

Table 1.1. A small portion of a typical data dictionary of variables and attributes for an EHR

Variable	Type	Length	SAS Format	Missing Data (%)	Description
Age	Numeric	8	8.1	0.4	Patient's age. Calculated using birth date and Encounter date and extracted from Patient and Demographic table.
Allergy	Character	255	$255.00	0	All patients' allergies from Allergy Intolerance table.
Allergy_Date	Numeric	8	MMDDYY10.	0	The date the allergy was first reported in Allergy Intolerance table.
Allergy_Severity	Character	255	$255.00	0	The severity of allergy reported in Allergy Intolerance table.
Birth_Date	Numeric	8	6.2	0.3	The date of birth for patients from Patient/Demographic tables.
BMI	Numeric	8	MMDDYY10.	3.2	Body Mass Index: kg/m2 from Exam table.
BMI_Date	Numeric	8	MMDDYY10.	3.2	Date that BMI in Exam table was recorded.
...	...	...	...	...	...
Vaccine	Character	255	$255.00	0	All vaccinations given to the patient using Vaccine table.
Vaccine_Date	Numeric	8	MMDDYY10.	0	The date that the vaccination was carried out.

1.5. Record Linkage

EHR tables and data sets often contain different information. Appropriate linking tables from the same EHR system is crucial to fully achieve the potential these data offer to research. Record linkage is commonly used to combine patient information from different tables within the same EHR and generate a comprehensive data set for analysis. Linkage increases the information by merging patient demographic data, symptoms and diseases, medications, laboratory results and other useful data, resulting in an increase in the dimension of the knowledge gained from EHR.

To combine two or more tables, you need to use unique and appropriate IDs that are common in the tables. Most EHR tables have more than one IDs. These IDs are unique for each patient, site or provider. For example, if you are planning to combine patient demographic information (sex, age) with prescribed medications then you should merge Patient or Demographic table with Medication table using Patient_ID. On the other hand, if you need to link billing information to healthcare provider or sites, then you should merge the Billing table with Provider or Site table using Provider_ID or Site_ID, respectively.

References

AHIMA. 2012. *Pocket Glossary of Health Information Management and Technology*, 3rd ed. Chicago, IL: AHIMA Press.

Ehsani-Moghaddam B., Martin K. and Queenan J. A. 2019. Data Quality in Healthcare: A Report of Practical Experience with CPCSSN Data. *Health Information Management Journal*. https://doi.org/10.1177/1833358319887743.

Electronic Health Record (EHR) Privacy and Security Requirements. 2005. Canada Health Infoway. https://www.infoway-inforoute.ca/en/component/edocman/389-ehr-privacy-and-security-requirements/view-document?Itemid=0.

HIMSS. Resource Center. http://www.himss.org/ASP/topics_ehr.asp.

Kruse C. S., Smith B., Vanderlinden H. and Nealand A. 2017. Security techniques for the electronic health records. *J Med Syst.* 41(8):127. https://doi.org/10.1007/s10916-017-0778-4.

OECD. 2017. "Data quality." In *OECD Handbook for Internationally Comparative Education Statistics: Concepts, Standards, Definitions and Classifications*. Paris: OECD Publishing. https://doi.org/10.1787/9789264279889-9-en.

Weiskopf, N. G., Bakken, S., Hripcsak, G., & Weng, C. (2017). A data quality assessment guideline for electronic health record data reuse. *EGEMs (Generating Evidence & Methods to Improve Patient Outcomes)*, 5(1), 14. https://doi.org/10.5334/egems.218.

Wickboldt A. K., Piramuthu S. 2012. Patient safety through RFID: Vulnerabilities in recently proposed grouping protocols. *J. Med. Syst.* 36(2):431–435. https://doi.org/10.1007/s10916-010-9487-y.

Chapter 2

Data Transfer from Database Management Systems to SAS

Abstract

Longitudinal healthcare records updates occur electronically over time for a population. To manage such records, many healthcare organizations now store data and manage data in relational databases. A relational database is a type of database that utilizes a structure that gives you access to data in relation to another piece of data in the database. In a relational database, data sets are often stored into tables. Connections between the tables are carried out using foreign keys. A foreign key, for example a Patient_ID, is a unique reference that can connect one row in a table to another row in another table. A relational database management system (RDBMS) is software that allows you to create, change and manage a relational database. Many relational database management systems use the SQL (Structured Query Language) to access the database. To get access to the database server and to establish a connection between SAS and the server, you may need to obtain permission from the database administrator and get authentication details.

In this chapter, you will be introduced to the three most popular RDBMSs. Then you will learn how to transfer EHR data from these data management systems to SAS program. For this chapter and the rest of book, except Chapter 11, SAS 9.4 TS Level 1M3 or later editions including SAS Enterprise Guide and SAS Studio can be used. For Chapter 11, SAS Enterprise Miner Workstation 15.1 or later edition must be used.

2.1. SQL Server

SQL Server is developed and marketed by Microsoft. Like other RDBMSs, SQL Server was created using SQL, a standard programming language to interact with relational databases. The main component of the SQL Server is the database engine, which includes a relational engine and a storage engine.

The relational engine processes queries and the storage engine manages database files. Currently, SQL Server works in both Windows environment and Linux. Microsoft offers two free SQL Server editions with different bundled services and tools:

- SQL Server Developer edition, which is a full-featured, licensed for use as a development and test database in a non-production environment.
- SQL Server Express, which is ideal for development and production for the desktop, the web, and small server applications and for databases with the size up to 10 GB (2014 edition).

2.1.1. How to Access a SQL Server Database from SAS

SAS provides several methods for extracting data from RDBMS and converting the data to SAS data sets. You can get access to the entire database and import individual SQL tables using either SAS/ACCESS Interface to Open Database Connectivity (ODBC) of Windows and PROC SQL or SAS/ACCESS to Object Linking and Embedding, Database (OLE DB). Here you are introduced to the SAS/ACCESS Interface to ODBC. For SAS/ACCESS Interface to OLEDB see the SAS technical paper in the References (Ref. 1). To obtain more information on how to download and install the ODBC driver see the SAS technical paper in the References (Ref. 2).

The process of importing the database using ODBC is easy and straight forward. The following steps can help you to get a connection between SAS and SQL Server:

1. Make sure the **sasioodb.dll** Access Interface file has been installed on your computer. This file is necessary to make the connection that you need. The default directory for this file is SASFoundation. For example:

   C:\Program Files\SASHome\SASFoundation\9.4\access\sasexe

2. Next, you need to set up an ODBC data source. In the search bar located on the left-hand side of your Windows taskbar type **ODBC**. This will bring you to the Data Source Administrator (Figure 2.1).

Data Transfer from Database Management Systems to SAS 17

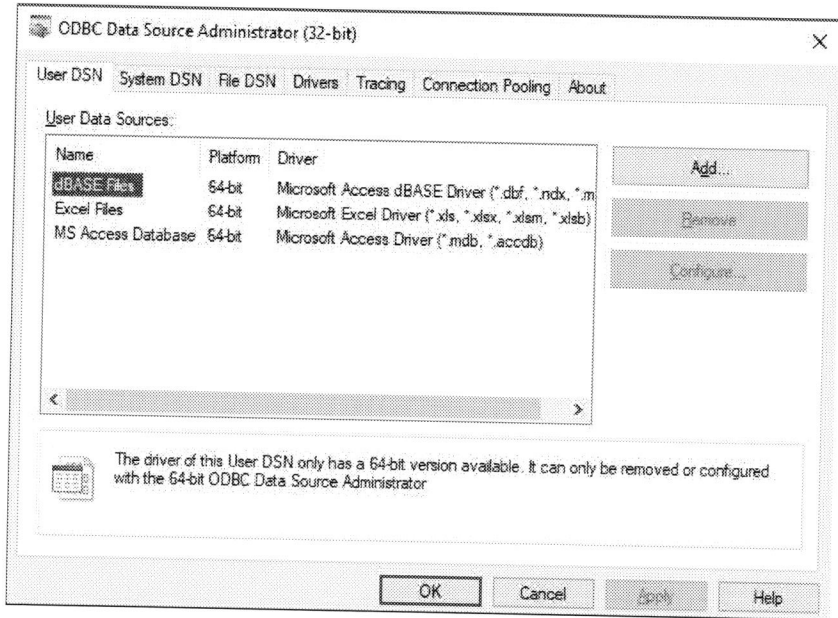

Figure 2.1. The ODBC data source.

3. Select the **User DSN** tab and then click on **Add** to add a new data source. Select the **SQL Server**. This will bring you the following wizard (Figure 2.2).

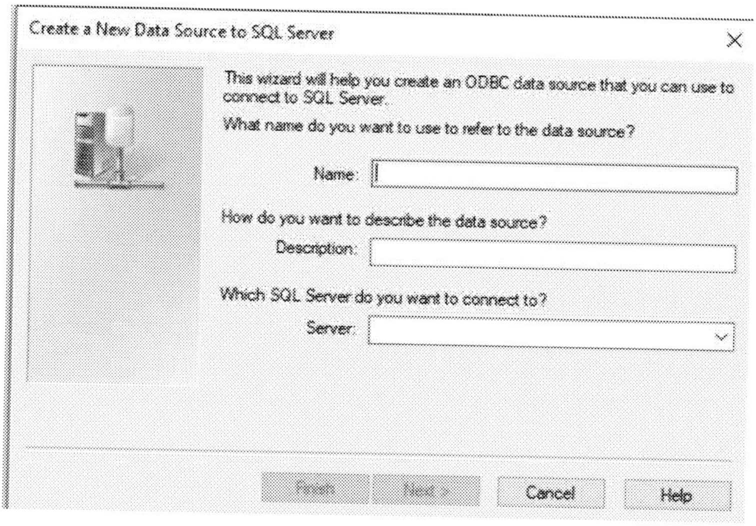

Figure 2.2. The wizard to create a data source.

Enter a name for your database and a brief description of the data (optional) and the server's name. Then click on **Next**. For this example, data source name is called **EHR_Database**.

4. SQL Server needs to know how to verify the authenticity of the login ID (Figure 2.3). You can either choose Windows authentication using the same ID that you always use to login into your computer or with SQL Server authentication. If you choose the first option, SQL Server is going to use your Windows-ID and password automatically and log into the server. Otherwise, if you choose the second option, then you need to create a login-ID and password.

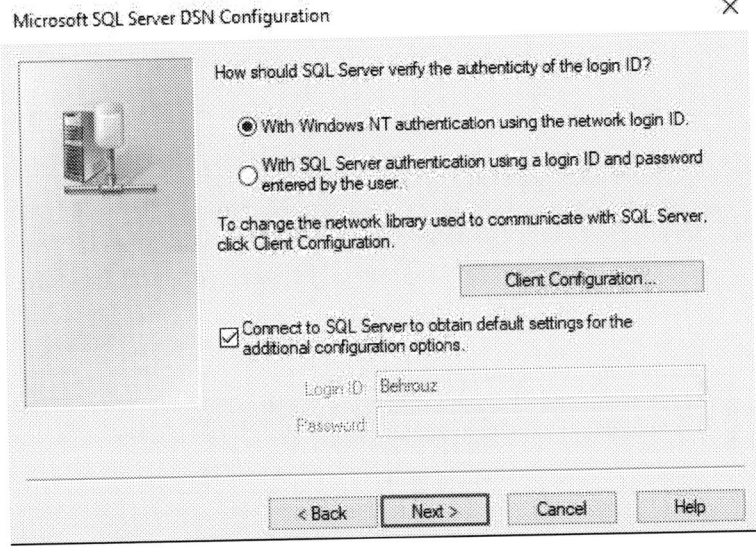

Figure 2.3. Verification of the authenticity by SQL Server.

Either way, by clicking on **Next**, you can go to the next step. In Figure 2.4, you can either configure the server such as changing the default database or changing the language of SQL server system messages, etc., or if you do not want to configure the server, you can escape this step and press the **Finish** tab.

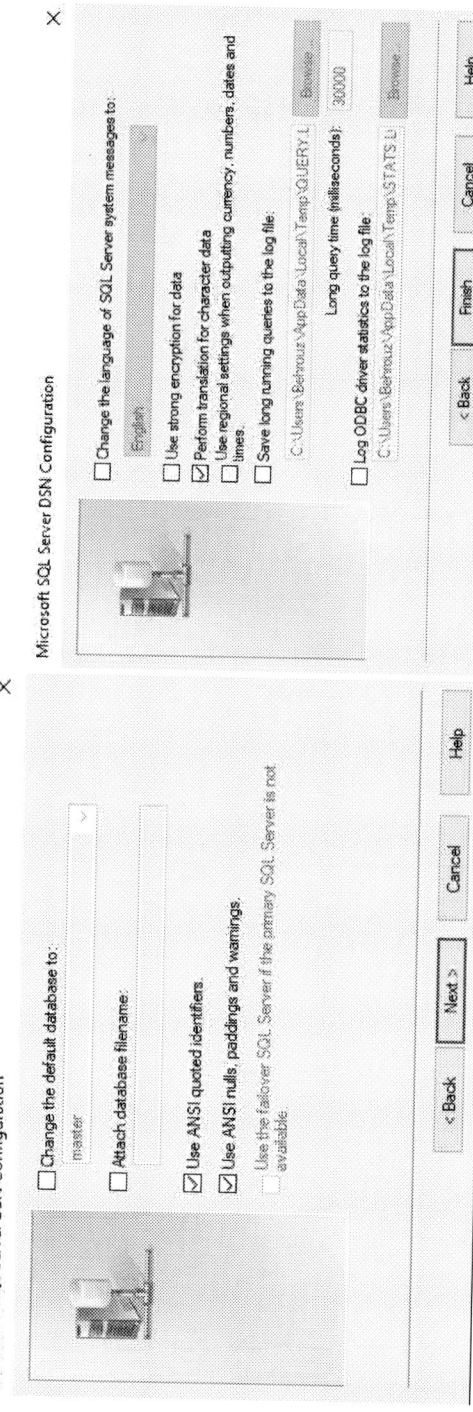

Figure 2.4. DSN configuration.

After clicking on the Finish tab, you will see the summary of the configurations you have applied. Before exiting the wizard, you can press the **Test** tab to see if the configurations are valid. If everything were carried out properly, you would see the following validation results (Figure 2.5).

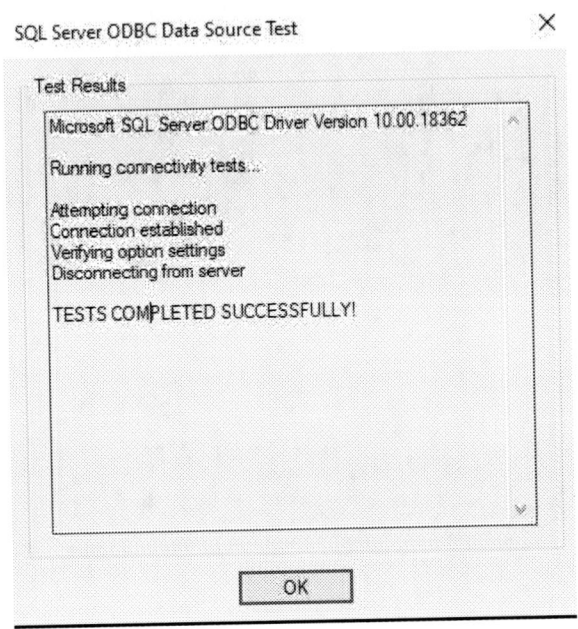

Figure 2.5. Test results of configurations in SQL server.

5. The last step is creating a SAS library for ODBC data source that you created using the following example codes:

Program 2.1. Creation of Libraries to Extract SQL Tables

```
libname Test odbc noprompt="dsn=EHR_database;
Trusted_Connection=yes" schema=dbo;
```

In the program 2.1, **Test** is the library name. In SAS, the **Libname** statement links the name of your library to the physical location of the library. The library names must be limited to eight characters, starting with a letter or underscore and contain only letters, numbers, or underscores. In the Test library, **dsn** denotes database name. Tables of databases in SQL Server are arranged in schemas. To see a particular table in a defined library, you may

Data Transfer from Database Management Systems to SAS

need to add the SCHEMA= option to the LIBNAME statement. Thus, the schema specifies a subfolder under the database. By adding schema=dbo to libname Test, the SQL Server tables will be visible in the SAS Explorer window.

During ODBC configuration, if you select SQL Server authentication, then you need to add the username and password to the libname **Test** in Program 2.1.

After running Program 2.1 and if creation of the library is set up properly, you will see the following message in the log:

```
libname Test odbc
noprompt=XXXXXXXXXXXXXXXXXXXXXXXXXXXXXXXXXXXXXXXXX
schema=DBO;

NOTE: Libref TEST was successfully assigned as follows:
      Engine:        ODBC
      Physical Name: EHR_database
```

2.1.2. Importing Individual EHR Tables

To extract individual data sets (tables) from SQL database or any other databases, you need to create another library. In Program 2.2, **EHR_Book** is the library name and the "C:\Users\...\Documents\EHR_Tables" statement denotes the physical location. **EHR_Tables** is the name of the folder that you have created before and is ready to store your SQL data sets. You can choose the location according to your preference.

Program 2.2. Creation of a Library to Extract SQL Tables

```
libname EHR_Book "C:\Users\...\Documents\EHR_Tables";
```

Once the new library is successfully assigned, you can use either DATA step or PROC SQL to import the individual tables into your new EHR_Book library. Program 2.3 shows how you can import, for example, the Medication table from **Test** database (Test.medication) into **EHR_Book** library using DATA step (the first section of the program) or PROC SQL (the second section of the program).

Program 2.3. Importing Individual EHR Tables

```
Options compress=yes reuse=yes; /*For reducing storage and
work space*/
data EHR_Book.medication;
set Test.medication;
quit;

Options compress=yes reuse=yes;
proc sql;
create table EHR_Book.medication as select*from
Test.medication;
quit;
```

2.2. Python

Python is an open source and a general-purpose programming language. Python supports data query statements, and data manipulation language, which make it an ideal language for database management. As a scripting language with simple syntax and rich text processing tools, Python is also used in artificial intelligence and natural language processing.

Perhaps, the easiest and simplest way to export data sets from Python to SAS is creating a data frame using the Pandas module of Python and then converting the data frame to CSV, or other flat files and then importing them directly into SAS using SAS Import Wizard or import program. In Program 2.4, for example, a data frame is created from Vaccine data (call it DataFrame), then it will be converted to CSV file in Python.

Program 2.4. Creating CSV File from Vaccine Data in Python

```
df = pd.DataFrame(vaccine, columns= ['Patient_ID', ...,
'Date_Created'])
print (df)
df.to_csv('C:\Users\...\Documents\EHR_Tables\export_da
taframe.csv')
```

In Program 2.4, 'Patient_ID', ..., 'Date_Created' are the name of columns. Then using SAS codes (Program 2.5), it will be imported into SAS.

Program 2.5. Importing CSV File Created in Python into SAS

```
proc import
datafile='C:\Users\...\Documents\EHR_Tables\dataframe.csv'
dbms=csv out=EHR_Book.Vaccine replace;
getnames=yes;
run;
```

In Program 2.5, **DATAFILE** shows the physical location of DataFrame. The **OUT** option denotes the name of data set that will be created and the SAS library name that the file will be located. The replace option will replace the new created file with the existing old file. The **GETNAMES=YES** tells SAS to use the column names. The type of file can be indicated by **DBMS**, which stands for Database Management Systems. For delimiter files it should be changed to **DBMS=DLM**. The created file can also be imported to SAS using Import Wizard and by clicking on File tab in SAS, then clicking on Import and then by simply following the steps (Figure 2.6).

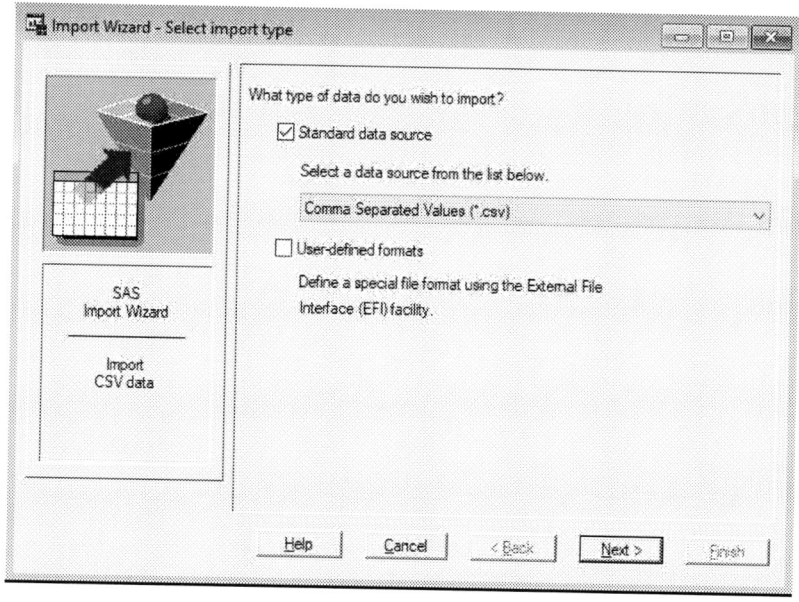

Figure 2.6. Data import wizard to import different types of data to SAS.

2.3. Oracle Healthcare Repository

Oracle Healthcare Data Repository is an inclusive data warehouse that allows patient, provider, and healthcare data across the healthcare organization to be unified and merged in a secure fashion. Oracle Healthcare Data Repository serves also as an operational data store and lets patient EHR information such as all encounters can easily be shared by authorized personnel across a healthcare organization. There are two SAS licenses that are needed and can be used to access Oracle database in the Windows environment as described in the SAS technical paper in the References (Ref. 3):

- SAS/ACCESS Interface to Oracle
- SAS/ACCESS Interface to ODBC

The SAS/ACCESS Interface provides support for the SQL Procedure Pass-Through Facility, which can be used to access data. The LIBNAME engine support for accessing data is also available to the SAS/ACCESS product. Accessing the database tables LIBNAME engine or PROC SQL is easy. If SAS/ACCESS has already been installed in the SAS server, you can use for example, Program 2.6 to connect to the database by LIBNAME engine (Example 1) or by PROC SQL (Example 2).

Program 2.6. Importing Oracle Tables into SAS

```
/* Example 1 */
libname mydblib oracle user=your_user_name
password=your_password path=path_to_database;

/* Example 2 */
proc sql;
connect to oracle
user=your user name orapw=Oracle password path=sample);
create table table-name as
select * from connection to oracle
(select * from data-name);
disconnect from oracle;
quit;
```

Similar to Section 2.1.2, once the new library is successfully created, the individual tables can be extracted into your new library (e.g., into EHR_Book library) using either a DATA step or PROC SQL (See Program 2.3.).

In addition to the SAS/ACCESS Interface to Oracle DBMS, the process of importing an Oracle database can be done using ODBC, as described before for SQL Server database (Section 2.1.1). To be able to use this method, you need to install the correct driver of ODBC for Oracle Client, if your system does not have it. Then you need to set up an ODBC data source that points to the database similar to the SQL Server in Section 2.1.1. Unlike ODBC, a pass-through SQL query processes data in its native environment using native SQL functions and moves processing operations closer to storage location. Since physical processing and storage locations impact processing speed, using pass-through SQL results in better efficiency, minimizes I/O operations, and reduces processing time. Furthermore, availability of certain functions to use in the RDBMS that are not supported by SAS is another advantage of using the pass-through SQL.

If your SAS server does not contain SAS/ACCESS, then you can first convert the individual tables to CSV or other flat files in Oracle. Then you can import the data sets into SAS using Program 2.5 or using Import Wizard as described before for SQL server databases in Section 2.2.

References

Parliyan A. *Getting Oracle Data into SAS® Datasets.* https://www.lexjansen.com/nesug/nesug02/ph/ph007.pdf.

Reiss M. Y., and Research W. 2020. *Extracting Data from Oracle® into SAS® Lessons Learned.* https://www.lexjansen.com/nesug/nesug04/io/io04.pdf.

SAS Communities Library. https://support.sas.com/techsup/technote/accessing-microsoft-sql-server-from-sas.pdf.

SAS OBC Drivers. User's Guide. https://support.sas.com/en/software/sas-odbc-drivers.html.

Chapter 3

Creating Temporary and Permanent Data Sets

Introduction

In Sections 2.1.1 and 2.1.2 in the previous chapter, you learned how to create a new library and how to import the individual data sets into your library. In this chapter, you will learn how to make temporary and permanent data sets, how to explore the EHR data sets, how to create subset data, and how to export the created data to other statistical programs. Learning these skills is necessary for success in analyzing data and for effective extraction of useful information from your database, which will be explained in the next chapters.

3.1. Making Temporary and Permanent Data Sets

In SAS you can analyze or process your data, but first you need to submit the data into a format that SAS can read it. There are several methods to submit your data into SAS and subsequently create data set.

1. You can use a DATA step and INPUT statement to put your data directly into a SAS program. This method is useful for a small data set. For example, in Program 3.1, by putting your data directly into the program you can make a data set. Since the name that is chosen for this data set (PatientVisit) is a one-level name and without any library name, SAS will create a temporary data set in the WORK library, which will exist only for the period of your current session and will be deleted at the end of session.

Program 3.1: Example of Creating a Data Set by Using DATA Step and INPUT Statement

```
data PatientVisit;
```

```
input Weight Visit Married Smoker;
datalines;
4111    1   1   0
3997    3   1   0
3572    3   1   0
1956    3   1   0
3515    3   1   0
3757    3   1   0
2977    3   0   1
3884    3   0   0
3629    3   1   0
3062    3   1   0
4026    3   1   1
3642    3   1   0
2296    3   .   0
2665    3   0   1
2948    3   1   0
3467    3   1   0
3430    3   1   0
4139    3   1   0
3657    .   1   0
3223    1   0   .
;
```

The PatientVisit data set has a rectangular shape with rows that are observations and columns that are variables including Weight, Visit, Married and Smoker. In SAS, keeping the rectangular shape of the data set is necessary. You can replace the missing observations with the dot to retain the rectangular shape as you see for the PatientVisit data set. You can also store the data set permanently, by adding a library name before the data set name for example: EHR_Book.PatientVisit. The library name must be the physical name for your SAS library. For more information about creating a new library, refer to Section 2.1.

2. You can create an identical (either temporary or permanent) data set using FILENAME and LIBNAME statements, and by using the DATA step. The FILENAME statement introduces an external file to SAS program, and the LIBNAME statement assigns a SAS data set or a DBMS file to the program. Program 3.2 shows you how to create a data set using either FILENAME or LIBNAME, and a DATA step or from another available data set. As you saw before, keeping the rectangular shape of data set is essential in SAS because for data sets that are created by these methods, SAS replaces

missing values for numeric variables with the dot and for character variables with blanks to retain the rectangular shape.

Program 3.2: Making Data Sets by FILENAME, LIBNAME or Another Data Set

```
/*Example 1*/
filename referral "c:\users\...\referral.dat";/*physical
address for your external data*/

libname ehr_book "c:\users\...\ehr_book";/*physical address for
your ehr_book library and sas file*/

/*Making a temporary data set from permanent data*/
data referral;
set ehr_book.referral;
run;

/*Example 2*/
/*Making a permanent data set from temporary data*/
data ehr_book.referral;
set referral;
run;
```

3.2. Exploring Your Data Set

After you connect your SAS to a database server and import a data set, it is always a good idea to get insight from the data set, investigate that the file was imported correctly, and the variables are those that you needed. Here you will be introduced to several methods to explore SAS data sets.

3.2.1. SAS Explorer

The first tool that you can use to get insight from your data and manage your data sets is the SAS Explorer. The SAS Explorer icon is in both on the toolbar and in the **View** tab. By clicking on the SAS Explorer icon and then on the library that you created for EHR database, you will find the data sets that were stored in the library. By double-clicking on an individual data set, the entire data set will be opened. You can also right-click on the data set and on the "Properties" of a pop-up menu to get access to some basic information such as date created or modified, number of columns and rows, and so on. More details about your data can be obtained by clicking on the **Details** or **View Columns** tab of the same pop-up menu.

3.2.2. CONTENTS Procedure

The contents of a data set can be explored by the CONTENTS procedure or by the CONTENTS statement of the DATASETS procedure. Both methods create metadata and variable information. The CONTENTS procedure provides information about an individual SAS dataset, whereas the CONTENTS and DATASETS procedures create information about the entire library and its data sets. There is no difference between these two methods except that for the CONTENTS procedure the default library is Work. By default, the CONTENTS procedure uses the most recently created SAS data set, unless you identify the data set. For the CONTENTS statement of the DATASETS procedure, the default is the libref of the procedure input library. For example, Program 3.3 can be used to obtain information from Sashelp.bmt (bone marrow transplant) data set, which is available in SAS Help folder.

Program 3.3: Contents View Using PROC CONTENTS and PROC DATASETS

```
proc datasets lib=Sashelp;
contents data=bmt;
run;

proc contents data=Sashelp.bmt out=info;
run;
```

Both programs print an alphabetical listing of the variable names by default. The results from the contents of Sashelp.bmt file gives you valuable information such as name, type, length, and label of the variables. According to the results of Program 3.3, the data set has 137 observations (rows) and three variables. One of the variables (Group) is character and the rest are numeric. The results of PROC CONTENTS can be stored in a new file, if you specify a file name (for example Info) for the output using "OUT" option.

3.2.3. PRINT Procedure

PROC PRINT invokes the PRINT procedure, which prints all or a subset of the observations in a SAS table. The reports can be a simple table or a highly customized report with grouping the data and calculating totals and subtotals of numeric variables. By default, PROC PRINT produces HTML reports when you run SAS in the Windows environment. For example, Program 3.4 prints the first 10 observations from the bone marrow transplant (bmt) data set. In the program, OBS=10 is an optional statement to view a certain number of rows. If you drop the statement, the program prints all observations. The title and footnote statements are also optional.

Program 3.4: Data Exploration Using PROC PRINT

```
proc print data=Sashelp.bmt (obs=10);
var group t;
title 'Bone Marrow Transplant';
footnote '*T: Disease-Free Survival Time';
run;
```

You can also change the style of print output by clicking on the following tabs:

Tools - Options - Preferences - Results - Style

3.2.4. FREQ Procedure

Another useful and very important method that you can use and discover basic information about your data sets is the FREQ procedure. The PROC FREQ statement invokes the procedure and by default, it uses the most recently created SAS data set, unless you identify the data set by Data=option. The FREQ procedure has many applications and options. For details, refer to the SAS/STAT user's guide. Using Program 3.5, you can get frequency and some other basic information about variables in the Framingham Heart Study data set. The data set is available in the SAS Help folder. In Program 3.5, the "ods graphics on" statement commands SAS to create a plot. ODS graphics remain active until you disable it with "ods graphics off" statement. The plots can be bar charts or dot plots. The ORDER=FREQ option orders the variables to appear by their frequency. The

NOCOL and NOROW options suppress the column and row percentages for each cell, respectively, and the CUMCOL option requests the cumulative column percentage for each cell.

Program 3.5: Data Exploration Using PROC FREQ

```
ods graphics on;
proc freq data=sashelp.heart order=freq;
tables chol_status*weight_status /
plots=freqplot(type=dotplot);
tables smoking_status/ nocol norow cumcol;
tables status/ nocol norow;
tables deathcause/ nocol norow cumcol;
title 'frequency of select variables in framingham heart
study';
run;
ods graphics off;
```

3.2.5. MEANS/SUMMARY Procedure

PROC MEANS and PROC SUMMARY are very efficient tools to provide basic statistics, information, and summary reports for numeric variables in a data set. You can obtain count (N), mean, median, mode, standard deviation, minimum and maximum, variance, standard error, number of missing data, range, quantile, and other information. The results can be saved as an output file if you use the OUTPUT option and identify a name for the file. These two procedures have the same capabilities. One of the primary differences between these two procedures is the way each one creates printed tables. By default, PROC MEANS always creates a table unless you use the NOPRINT option. In contrast, the SUMMARY procedure never creates a printed table unless you use the PRINT option to request printing the table.

Program 3.6 shows you how to use PROC MEANS and PROC SUMMARY to get useful information about diastolic and systolic blood pressure of the Framingham Heart Study data. In both parts of this program, N, MEAN, MAX, MIN, RANGE, STD, CLM, and MAXDEC correspond to the number of observations, mean, maximum value, minimum value, range of data (difference between the highest and the lowest values), standard deviation, two-sided 95% confidence limits, and maximum number after decimal, respectively. As you see from the program, the only difference between Example 1 and Example 2 of the program is the BY statement.

Creating Temporary and Permanent Data Sets

Here, using the BY statement can classify the results for sex (Table 3.1). When you use the BY option, the input data must be sorted by the classes of BY variables prior to running the codes, otherwise you will see an error message. When you are using a big data set with many observations, even if the BY statement is not used, sorting data prior to running PROC MEANS or PROC SUMMARY can help you to minimize the processing time.

Program 3.6: Data Exploration Using PROC MEANS and PROC SUMMARY

```
/*Example 1: without By statement*/
data heart; /*you need to make a new data, because available
data in sashelp folder cannot be sorted or manipulated. let's
call the new data set heart*/
set sashelp.heart;

proc means data=heart n mean max min range std clm maxdec=1;
var diastolic systolic ;
title 'Diastolic And Systolic Information From Framingham Heart
Study';
run;

proc summary data=heart print n mean max min range std clm
maxdec=1;
var diastolic systolic ;
title 'Diastolic And Systolic Information From Framingham Heart
Study';
run;

/*Example 2: with By statement*/
proc sort data=heart;
by sex;
proc means data=heart n mean max min range std clm maxdec=1;
var diastolic systolic ;
by sex;
title 'Diastolic and Systolic By Sex for Framingham Heart
Study';
run;

proc summary data=heart print n mean max min range std clm
maxdec=1;
var diastolic systolic ;
by sex;
title 'Diastolic and Systolic By Sex for Framingham Heart
Study';
run;
```

Table 3.1. Diastolic and systolic by sex for Framingham Heart Study Data.

Sex=Female								
Variable	N	Mean	Maximum	Minimum	Range	Std Dev	Lower 95% CL for Mean	Upper 95% CL for Mean
Diastolic	2873	84.6	155.0	50.0	105.0	13.3	84.2	85.1
Systolic	2873	136.9	300.0	82.0	218.0	26.0	135.9	137.8
Sex=Male								
Variable	N	Mean	Maximum	Minimum	Range	Std Dev	Lower 95% CL for Mean	Upper 95% CL for Mean
Diastolic	2336	86.2	160.0	50.0	110.0	12.5	85.7	86.7
Systolic	2336	136.9	276.0	90.0	186.0	20.7	136.1	137.8

3.2.6. UNIVARIATE Procedure

One of the most useful methods for exploring data and summarizing information is using the UNIVARIATE procedure. In this procedure, you can use the VAR statement to specify the numeric variables that needs to be analyzed. If the VAR statement is not defined, then all available numeric variables will be analyzed. By using the OUTPUT statement, you can save summary statistics in an output data set. You can also create different graphs such as PPPLOT, QQPLOT, and so on using the PLOT statement. You can also get group analyses if you use BY statement. If you use a CLASS statement to specify categorical variables, then SAS analyzes data based on the levels of class variables.

Program 3.7 shows you how to get univariate statistics including PPPLOT for systolic blood pressure of the Framingham Heart Study data for both female and male patients. By requesting PPPLOT (probability-probability plot), you can investigate the distribution of systolic observations and compare it with a known cumulative distribution function such as Normal. For example, you can compare it with a normal distribution with mean ($\mu=140$) and standard deviation ($\sigma=30$). If you do not specify μ and σ, the sample mean, and standard deviation will be used instead. The SQUARE option in the program displays the plots in a square layout.

Program 3.7: Data Exploration Using PROC UNIVARIATE

```
ods graphics on;
proc univariate data=sashelp.heart;
var systolic;
class sex;
ppplot systolic / normal(mu=140 sigma=30)square
odstitle = "Normal Distribution for Systolic Blood Pressure";
run;
ods graphics off;
```

3.3. Creating a Subset of Data

EHR data contains variables or information that are not always required for a particular research project or a particular analysis, in which case you might want to change the data set to contain only variables of interest. Furthermore, SAS programs run more quickly and occupy less storage space if data sets have only necessary variables. Data subsetting can be done in the variable (column or data element), observation (row), or in a character string level. In this section, you will learn how to select variables and subset data using the KEEP and DROP options in the DATA step or as statement, and how to subset data using IF, WHERE, and DELETE statements. Additionally, other useful methods are going to be explained as well. For the practical experience of this part, you will use the sashelp.heart data set.

3.3.1. KEEP and DROP Statements

In a DATA step, there are two methods of using KEEP and DROP to manipulate a data set: 1. DATA step statement; 2. Data set option. SAS DATA step statements begin with a keyword and end with a semicolon. Whereas data set option is applied in parentheses next to a data set. Heart data set that you created before for section 1.1.5 contains 17 variables. Suppose for your analysis, you only need the following variables:

- Status
- DeathCause
- AgeCHDdiag
- Sex

- AgeAtStart
- Height
- Weight
- Diastolic
- Systolic
- MRW

Using any of those examples in Program 3.7, you can achieve this goal. If you use the same data set name (Heart) for creating subset data, then SAS will substitute the new data set with the original one. If you need to keep the original data set, then you should use another name (e.g., Heart_1) for the subset data. The KEEP option/statement specifies which variables (columns) must be kept in a subset data, while the DROP option/statement specifies which variables must be excluded. The data set options are more flexible than the DATA step statements. For example, in Program 3.7, the KEEP and the DROP options can be applied in the data set being written (Example 1 and 4), the data set being read (Example 2 and 5), or both. In terms of program efficiency, Examples 2 and 5 are more efficient, because both KEEP and DROP options are applied to the program before the data are read into the DATA step.

Program 3.7: Subsetting Data Using KEEP and DROP

```
/*Example 1: Using Keep in data set option*/
data heart_1(keep=status deathcause agechddiag sex ageatstart
height weight diastolic systolic mrw);
set sashelp.heart;
run;

/*Example 2: Using Keep in data set option*/
data heart_1;
set sashelp.heart (keep=status deathcause agechddiag sex
ageatstart height weight diastolic systolic mrw);
run;

/*Example 3: Using Keep in DATA step statement*/
data heart_1;
set sashelp.heart;
keep status deathcause agechddiag sex ageatstart height weight
diastolic systolic mrw;
run;
```

```
/*Example 4: Using Drop in data set option */
data heart_1 (drop=smoking ageatdeath cholesterol chol_status
bp_status weight_status smoking_status);
set sashelp.heart;
run;

/*Example 5: Using Drop in data set option */
data heart_1;
set sashelp.heart(drop=smoking ageatdeath cholesterol
chol_status bp_status weight_status smoking_status);
run;

/*Example 6: Using drop in DATA step statement*/
data heart_1;
set sashelp.heart;
drop smoking ageatdeath cholesterol chol_status bp_status
weight_status smoking_status;
run;
```

3.3.2. Subsetting Data with PROC SQL

Similar to KEEP and DROP, you can keep or drop columns and subset data using PROC SQL. For example, in Program 3.8, PROC SQL can be used to create a subset of data (Heart_1) that includes only Status, DeathCause, AgeCHDdiag, Sex and Height variables.

Program 3.8: Subsetting Data Using PROC SQL

```
proc sql;
create table heart_1 as select status, deathcause, agechddiag,
sex, height from sashelp.heart;
quit;
```

3.3.3. Subsetting Using IF/WHERE/IF…THEN DELETE

IF/WHERE expressions can be used to specify which observations (*rows*) to be retained in a data set. Consider Example 1 in Program 3.9, the program creates a temporary subset data (Heart_1), which will be identical to sashelp.heart, except it will include records from female patients only with height values between 55 and 65 and without any missing observations for DeathCause and AgeCHDdiag variables. Unlike IF/WHERE statement, the

IF...THEN DELETE statement removes the observations that do not meet a specific condition. In Example 2 of Program 3.9, the conditional statement deletes observations that contain a missing value for DeathCause or AgeCHDdiag variables. Notice, since DeathCause is a character variable, the missing values are coded by "" instead of a dot (.).

Program 3.9: Subsetting Data Using IF/WHERE/IF... THEN DELETE

```
/*Example 1*/
data heart_1;
set sashelp.heart;
if sex="female" and 55<height<65 and deathcause not eq "" and
agechddiag not eq .;
run;
data heart_1;
set sashelp.heart;
where sex="female" and 55<height<65 and deathcause not eq ""
and agechddiag not eq .;
run;

/*example 2*/
data heart_1;
set sashelp.heart;
if deathcause eq "" or agechddiag=. then delete;
run;
```

3.3.4. Subsetting Data Using CONTAINS, LIKE, FIND, INDEX and SUBSTR Functions

As you may have noticed before, subset data can be created by keeping or dropping columns or rows. Sometimes during analysis of EHR data, you need to subset data based on some specific criteria, for example a specific observation or character strings. SAS has several functions such as CONTAINS, LIKE, INDEX, and SUBSTR, which can help you. Both CONTAINS and LIKE functions can be used with WHERE in a DATA step to search a character variable for a specified string. They both are case sensitive and select rows by comparing character strings with a specified pattern that is matched. For example, suppose in sashelp.heart you need to create a subset of data (call it Heart_1) that, you only need those records,

Creating Temporary and Permanent Data Sets

which their DeathCause column has "Cerebral Vascular Disease." Examples 1 and 2 from Program 3.10 show you how to make such data.

LIKE can also be used in conjunction with "%" as the wildcard to perform keyword search for character variables that start/end/contain certain character strings (see example 3 of Program 3.10). To obtain the comparable result in an IF statement, the FIND and INDEX functions can be used. The FIND operator can be applied with the 'i' argument to ignore case. The INDEX function searches a character string (a character constant, variable, or expression), from left to right, for the first occurrence of the specified string of characters and has two arguments, source (variable name) and excerpt (character string or expression). Like the INDEX function, the FIND function also searches for the first occurrence of the specified substring of characters in a character string; nevertheless, unlike INDEX it has a modifier and a start-position argument. If start-position is not specified, the search starts at the beginning of the string from left to right. For example, you might need your subset to include only those observations whose "Chol_Status" records contain "Borderline." Both Example 4 and 5 from Program 3.10 will give you the subset that you need.

Finally, the SAS DATA step SUBSTRING (SUBSTR) function operates on character strings. SUBSTR returns a specified part of the input character string, starting at the position that is specified by user and can continue either side of the "=" sign. The SUBSTR function has three arguments: a SOURCE, which can be a variable or a string of characters; a POSITION, which is the starting point for reading the internal group of characters; and N, which is the number of characters or length to read from the starting point: SUBSTR (SOURCE, POSITION, N).

Suppose in sashelp.heart you need to subset data according to smoking habits of patients and you only need the records of those who are the non-smoker. Example 6 from Program 3.10 shows you how to get the subset using SUBSTR.

Program 3.10: Subsetting Data Using CONTAINS, LIKE, FIND, INDEX and SUBSTR Functions

```
/*Example 1*/
data heart_1;
set sashelp.heart;
where0 deathcause contains "cerebral vascular disease";
run;
```

```
/*Example 2*/
data heart_1;
set sashelp.heart;
where deathcause like "cerebral vascular disease";
run;

/*Example 3*/
data heart_1;
set sashelp.heart;
where deathcause like "cerebral%";
run;

/*Example 4*/
data heart_1;
set sashelp.heart;
if find(chol_status, "borderline","i");/*"i" is a modifier,
which can be used to ignore character case*/
run;

/*Example 5*/
data heart_1;
set sashelp.heart;
if index(chol_status, "borderline");
run;

/*Example 6*/
data heart_1;
set sashelp.heart;
if substr(smoking_status, 1, 3)="non";
run;
```

3.4. Exporting Data from SAS to Other Programs

You can easily export your SAS data sets to Microsoft® Excel, R, SPSS, STATA, and other programs. The created file can be exported to these programs using the Export Wizard and by clicking on the **File** tab in SAS, then clicking on **Export** and then by simply following the steps. There are also many other alternative ways, particularly for exporting data into Excel. In Program 3.11, for example, the temporary Heart_1 data set created from Program 3.10, which is located in Work library, is exported under different name (Heart_2) as tab-separated file, CSV, XLS, SPSS and STATA using PROC EXPORT. The REPLACE option replaces the new file with the old one.

Creating Temporary and Permanent Data Sets

Program 3.11: Exporting SAS Data Sets to Other Programs

```
/*Tab-separated file*/
proc export data=heart_1 outfile="physical address of the new
data\heart_2.txt" dbms=tab replace;
run;

/*CSV file*/
proc export data=heart_1 outfile="physical address of the new
data \heart_2.csv" dbms=csv replace;
run;

/*Excel (XLS) file*/sheet="Heart_1";
proc export data=heart_1 outfile="physical address of the new
data \heart_2" dbms=excel replace;
run;

/*SPSS file*/
proc export data= heart_1 outfile="physical address of the new
data \heart_2" dbms=sav replace;
run;

/*STATA file*/
proc export data= heart_1 outfile="physical address of the new
data \heart_2" dbms=dta replace;
run;
```

Chapter 4

Retrieving Patient Information

Abstract

Using EHR data created during healthcare practice for research purposes is referred to as a secondary use of data because the data were primarily collected as part of routine patient care and not for research. That is why EHR data are profoundly different than other research data such as, for example, prospectively collected records of randomized controlled clinical trials. Some of the major differences between EHR data and the data collected from clinical controlled trials are the lack of actual control over quality and quantity of observations, data collection processes, type of variables, and dependency on record linkage from one EHR data set to another. On the one hand, EHR data sets contain data elements that are unnecessary for research projects, and on the other hand, the information that is buried in one single table may not be enough. Understanding how to handle EHR data and do some basic tasks such as linking several different EHR tables into one single data set to obtain maximum useful information from patients, create new variables, and properly remove duplicate observations are fundamental for appropriate analysis of patient information.

Upon finishing this chapter, you will be able to combine two or more EHR tables to create a single data set with more useful variables or observations, remove unnecessary duplicate data, create new variables, change date format, calculate patient age from date of birth, and convert variable type from numeric to character or vice versa. At the end of this chapter, you will also be familiar with patient encounter date and its importance for analytics, and the necessity to create a comprehensive encounter date that covers all other EHR dates. The EHR database used for this, and the next chapters contain the following 12 SAS tables:

- Allergy (intolerance)
- Billing
- Encounter
- Encounter diagnosis
- Exam
- Health condition (problem list)

- Medication
- Patient
- Referral
- Risk factor
- Vaccine
- Vaers

These data sets, which have been artificially created for this book and the related data dictionary, are freely available to download from GitHub[1].

To better understand the concepts discussed in each chapter, it is highly advisable that you download all these data sets, then create a SAS library and name it **EHRData**. Use the data sets practically for the programs that are given during each chapter. Except for the Vaers data set, none of the information including Patient_IDs presented in these tables are real, and there is no connection between these artificial data sets with any actual EHR data sets. The source of information for Vaers data set will be discussed in Chapter 5.

4.1. Combining EHR Data Sets

In an EHR database, patient information such as demographic data and International Classification of Disease (ICD) codes are distributed across multiple tables. Often you need to combine these tables to retrieve the maximum amount of information from patients or to reduce the number of missing records. This section explains the most useful combining techniques for EHR tables. For a comprehensive method of combining or merging data sets, you can refer to Step-by-Step Programming with Base SAS® 9.4, Second Edition. Cary, NC: SAS Institute Inc. or Malachy J. Foley's paper titled "MERGING vs. JOINING: Comparing the DATA Step with SQL" (2009).

4.1.1. Concatenation

Combining two or more data sets into one single data set using a SET statement is called concatenation. By using this technique, you can add the contents of one data set to another one. The final product of the

---

[1] https://github.com/ebehrouz/SAS-Programming-for-Healthcare-Data.

concatenation in terms of number of observations and variables is the summation of all original data sets. In product of the concatenation, all observations from the first SAS tables are sequentially followed by all observations from the second data set, and so on. In case one of data sets contains different variables, the product will contain missing observations from the data set that does not have any value for those variables. Figure 4.1 illustrates the Venn diagram of a data set that is the product of combining the Billing table with 71,115 observations and the HealthCondition table with 71,115 observations from the EHRData database. The product of this concatenation has 142,230 observations.

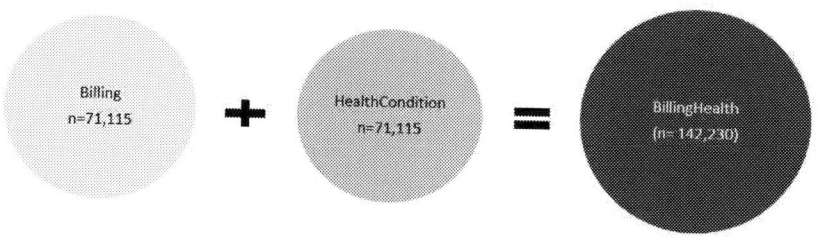

Figure 4.1. Venn diagram of combining two EHR data sets using concatenation.

You can use Program 4.1 and the SET statement to concatenate those two data sets.

Program 4.1: Example of Creating Data Set by Using a DATA Step and SET Statement

```
data BillingHealth;
     set ehrdata.billing ehrdata.healthcondition;
run;
```

The BillingHealth data set created from Program 4.1 is not arranged by any variable. If you need the observations to be arranged by the values of a variable, you can do so by sorting the data first and then using the BY variable(s). The new data set will be a combination of all other data sets and will be arranged by the BY group and by the order of the data sets that they occur. Program 4.2 shows you how to combine those two data sets from Program 4.1 by the DiagnosisCode_calc variable. The concatenation method that uses the BY statement is called interleaving.

Program 4.2: Example of Creating Data Set Using BY and Interleaving Method

```
proc sort data=ehrdata.billing;
      by diagnosiscode_calc;

proc sort data=ehrdata.healthcondition;
      by diagnosiscode_calc;

data billinghealth;
      set ehrdata.billing ehrdata.healthcondition;
      by diagnosiscode_calc;
run;
```

4.1.2. Match-Merging

Sorting two or more data sets by a common key variable (ID) and matching them up into one single output file is called match-merging. Consider the same two EHRData tables from Section 4.1.1. They can be combined using their common key-ID (Patient_ID) to produce seven different data sets. The Venn diagram in Figure 4.2 and Program 4.3 illustrate all seven possible combinations of these two data sets.

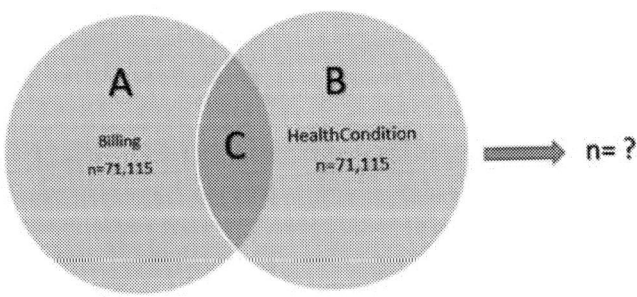

Figure 4.2. Venn diagram of combining two EHR data sets using ID and match-merging technique.

The question mark in Figure 4.2 denotes the fact that, unlike combining data sets by concatenation, the number of observations in the product of merging technique is not always predictable depending on conditional statements of the program. Therefore, when you combine data sets using match-merging technique you should always be cautious because it can produce undesirable results. As such, you need to test your program on samples of the data sets and the product of merging before using this method to combine the main data sets.

Consider the Billing table as A and the HealthCondition table as B and the subset of data, which is common in these two data sets as C. Program 4.3 uses the same input files as Program 4.1, but because of using conditional statements, there would be seven different output files.

Program 4.3: Example of Creating Data Sets Using Match-Merging Technique

```
proc sort data=ehrdata.billing;
      by Patient_ID;
run;

proc sort data=ehrdata.healthcondition;
      by Patient_ID;
run;

data AC BC C A_Only B_Only ABC AB;
      merge ehrdata.billing(in=A)
ehrdata.healthcondition(in=B);
      by patient_id;

      if A=1 then
            output AC;

      if B=1 then
            output BC;

      if (A=1 and B=1) then
            output C;

      if (A=1 and B=0) then
            output A_Only;

      if (A=0 and B=1) then
            output B_Only;

      if (A=1 or B=1) then
            output ABC;

      if (A+B)=1 then
            output AB;
run;
```

In Program 4.3, data from both the Billing and HealthCondition tables are sorted by Patient_ID first, then they are merged in different ways. Patient_ID is a foreign identification key, which is common and consistent for each patient across different EHR data sets and can be utilized to link one table to another one. In Table 4.1, the concept of each merge has been described as fully understanding that Program 4.3 is essential for all further data manipulation and analysis. The output file ABC is the default match-merge, which contains all information from both of data sets. Other output data sets are subsets of ABC, which can be created by conditional statement of "IF ...THEN" and 1 and 0 (1 for the present of data and 0 for otherwise).

Table 4.1. Description of data sets created by match-merging

Data Set*	Description
AC	Records in A including those common with B
BC	Records in B including those common with A
C	Only records that are common between A and B
A_Only	Records in A that are not common with B
B_Only	Records in B that are not common with A
ABC	All records from both A and B including common records
AB	All records from A and B except those that are common between A and B

* A=Billing table, B= HealthCondition table, and C=common records from A and B.

Some of these data sets in Table 4.1 (BC, B_Only, ABC, and AB) can also be created using PROC SQL, which the product is called a join. The SQL procedure and the DATA step use completely different method to combine data sets, consequently the products from a match-merge and a join are often different. PROC SQL can reproduce the match-merge results in four cases out of seven possible combinations of Table 4.1 with some limitations such as the full and right joins need to use the COALESCE function or some other alternative codes.

4.2. Creating New Variables

During EHR analysis, very often you may need to create a new variable. The new variable can be created without any need for other variables or from other available variables, as well.

4.2.1. Creating New Variables Using LENGTH or ATTRIB Statements

In Program 4.4, a temporary data set (Example) is created from EHRdata.Billing with two new variables, COPD and Diabetes, in the DATA step using LENGTH and ATTRIB statements, respectively. When you are using the LENGTH statement to create a new variable, it should be placed at the beginning in the DATA step before any other statements. As you see in Program 4.4, you can also use the ATTRIB statement together with LENGTH, FORMAT, or INFORMAT options to create a new variable.

Program 4.4: Example of Creating Variable Using LENGTH or ATTRIB Statements

```
data example;
      length COPD $25;
      set ehrdata.billing;
      COPD="No";
      attrib Diabete length=3;
      Diabete=1;
run;
```

4.2.2. Creating New Variables from Existing Variables

New variables can be created from other variables too. In Program 4.5, several examples are shown. In Example 1, a new variable called Mollaret is created using the HealthCondition and Patient tables of EHRData. This variable can be used to identify patients with Mollaret disease, a special type of meningitis due to a viral infection (aseptic meningitis). In the first section of the same example, two temporary data sets are created from the Patient and the HealthCondition tables, then they are sorted by Patient_ID. Meanwhile, DateOfOnset of the disease is converted to a SAS format for subsequent age estimation in Example 2. In the second section of Example 1, the created data sets are merged using match-merging which was discussed in Section 4.1.2. The data set that is created by merging technique is called Patient_healthcondition. In the third section of the same example, all patients who have ICD-10 code equal to "G032" in their DiagnosisCode_calcs, their Mollaret value will be equal to 1, otherwise it will be 0.

In Example 2, a new variable, which is called Anticoagulant is created from the Medication table of EHRData library. Those patients who have any of Heparin, Rivaroxaban, Warfarin, Dabigatran, Edoxaban drugs in their records (name_calc) of Medication table are going to have an Anticoagulant equal to 1, otherwise 0.

Program 4.5: Example of Creating Variables Using Existing Variables

```
/*Example 1*/
data patient;/*1*/
   set ehrdata.patient;
run;

proc sort data=patient;
   by patient_id;
run;

data healthcondition;
   set ehrdata.healthcondition;
      format dateofonset mmddyy10.;
run;

proc sort data=healthcondition;
   by patient_id;
run;

data patient_healthcondition;/*2*/

   merge patient(in=A) healthcondition(in=B);
     by patient_id;

     if A=1 then output patient_healthcondition;

run;

data patient_healthcondition;/*3*/

   set patient_healthcondition;

     if DiagnosisCode_calc="G032" then Mollaret=1;
     else Mollaret=0;

run;
```

Sorting data and making a new data set from another data can be done at the same time.

For example, the first section of Example 1 can be written as:

```
/*4*/
proc sort data=ehrdata.patient
                out=patient;
   by patient_id;
run;



/*Example 2*/
data medication;

  set ehrdata.medication;

    if name_calc in
("heparin","rivaroxaban","warfarin","dabigatran","edoxaban")
then Anticoagulant=1;
else Anticoagulant=0;
run;
```

4.3. Removing Duplicate or Unnecessary Records

Duplicate medical records are defined as two or more health record numbers assigned for a single patient at the same healthcare facility (Harris and Houser, 2018). For analytical purposes, the identification of duplicate observations (rows) or unnecessary records should be done proactively by understanding the nature of duplicate records and with regard to the scope of research project. Thus, before duplicates are removed, you need to investigate if removal is necessary or permitted. For example, routine BMI recording in EHR could help healthcare providers in the management of overall patient's health. Depending on the objectives of research project, multiple BMI records for each patient may be allowed to stay in the data set for final analysis or might not be necessary and need to be removed. In this section, you will be introduced to different approaches to remove duplicate or unwanted observations through several examples. But how can you figure out that the data that you are working on has duplicated observations? You can use the first section of Program 4.6 to see if EHRData.Exam has any duplicate data based on Patient_ID or not. If the program finds more than one observation for each Patient_ID, the output will be printed, otherwise there will be no print.

4.3.1. Example 1

Sometimes you only need to keep one observation for each patient and remove the rest of them regardless of the values of variables. For example, suppose you need to know the number of patients in the Exam table of EHRData. In the second section of Program 4.6, first you create a temporary data set (Exam) from the Exam data set (optional), then you sort data by Patient_ID, then you remove all observations except one of them, and at the end using PROC CONTENTS you can get the number of patients. By using a FIRST. statement, SAS creates a temporary variable. If the value of this temporary variable indicates that an observation is the first one in a BY group (by Patient_ID), then the conditional action will happen (here running the Exam data set).

Program 4.6: Example of Removing Duplicate or Unwanted Observations

```
/*1*/
data ehrdata.exam;
        set ehrdata.exam;
        count + 1;
        by patient_id;

        if first. patient_id then
                count=1;
run;

proc print;
        where count ge 2;
run;

/*2*/
data exam;
        set ehrdata.exam;
run;

proc sort data=exam;
        key patient_id;
run;

Data exam;
        Set exam;
        by patient_id;
```

```
        if first. patient_id;
run;

proc contents data=exam;
run;
```

4.3.2. Example 2

Suppose you are interested in knowing the frequency of patients with unspecified malignant neoplasm of colon (ICD-10 code: C189) in the entire EHRData. To determine the frequency of the disease, you need first to combine all records from the HealthCondition, Billing, and Encounter Diagnosis tables, then create a dummy variable called MNC. Those patients who have the code in their DiagnosisCode_calc variable get 1 and those without the code get 0 for MNC. Next, you need to sort data for Patient_ID either by DESCENDING or ASCENDING, and MNC by the DESCENDING option. The DESCENDING statement will sort the MNC variable from the highest (1) to the lowest (0) values for each patient. Then the NODUPKEY option keeps the first observation for each patient and drops the rest. Then the frequency of the disease can be obtained by FREQ procedure (Program 4.7).

Program 4.7: Example of Removing Duplicate Disease Data

```
data all;
        set ehrdata.healthcondition ehrdata.billing
ehrdata.encounterdiagnosis;

data all;
        set all;

        if diagnosiscode_calc="C189" then
                MNC=1;
        else
                MNC=0;
run;

proc sort data=all nodupkey;
        key patient_id MNC/descending;
run;
```

```
proc freq data=all;
      table MNC;
run;
```

4.3.3. Example 3

In this example, you need to keep the first (oldest) measurement for the repeated weight values from patients in the Exam table of EHRData and remove the rests. To do so, first you create a temporary data set (optional) from EHRData.Exam, then you sort data according to PerformedDate and Patient_ID from the oldest to the newest record by implementing an ASCENDING statement. Then you keep the first record only by dropping the extra observations (Program 4.8).

Program 4.8: Example of Removing Unwanted Repeated Weight Values

```
data exam;
      set ehrdata.exam;
run;

proc sort data=exam;
      key patient_id performeddate/ascending;
run;

Data exam;
      Set exam;
      by patient_id;

      if first. patient_id;
run;
```

4.4. Changing Date Format

Calendar dates may appear in a variety of formats in EHR tables. To be able to apply some basic operations such as addition, subtraction, and comparison, the calendar dates need to be converted to SAS format. SAS dates equal or after January 1, 1960, can be used for all types of analytical procedures. Dates before this date are handled as negative numbers by SAS. Although SAS software can read two-digit or four-digit year values, whenever possible, you should use a four-digit year. Otherwise, to appropriately handle two-digit years for dates between 2000 and 2099, you require an appropriate adjustment between 1901 and 2000 using YEARCUTOFF=.[2]

A SAS date value is a numeric variable. By using a FORMAT statement, you can indicate to SAS that the variable that is going to be used is a date. If a date value is printed by PROC PRINT without a FORMAT statement, it has appeared as the number of days since Jan 1, 1960. FORMAT can also be used to convert data to any desired permanent SAS date format. For example, DateCreated in EHRdata.Encounter data set has DATE9. format (e.g., 25JUN2016). To change this format to mmddyy10. (e.g., 06/25/2016), you can use Example 1 in Program 4.9. To create a constant SAS date as a cutoff date, make the date enclosed in single or double quotes, followed by a d. In Example 2 of Program 4.9, June 30th, 2018, is used as a cutoff point to subset records from the Exam table that were recorded after this date.

Program 4.9: Changing Date Format

```
/*Example 1*/
data encounter;
      set ehrdata.encounter;
      format DateCreated mmddyy10.;
run;

/*Example 2*/
data exam;
      set ehrdata.exam;
      where '30jun2018'd < datecreated;
run;
```

4.5. Estimation of Patient Age

Age for patients at the time of onset of a disease or at any other point can be computed using Program 4.10. To estimate patient age at the time of other occasions, other cutoff dates can be used such as ServiceDate, DateCreated and so on. In Program 4.10, you use the Patient_healthcondition data set

---

[2] For more information about how to read two-digit years using YEARCUTOFF= option and available SAS date formats refer to Step-by-Step Programming with Base SAS® 9.4, Second Edition. Cary, NC: SAS Institute Inc.

from Program 4.5. First, you add the Age variable to the Patient_healthcondition data set, then you create Birthdate variable from BirthDay, BirthMonth, and BirthYear. As mentioned earlier, the DateOfOnset needs to be converted to SAS format (mmddyy10.). In the Program 4.10, the FORMAT age 6.1 statement makes the calculated age with one digit after the decimal, the unnecessary variables are dropped from the data set, and if in a data set, the birthdate variable is in a single column and includes birthday, birth month, and birth year, then the following equation and code is not necessary in the first section and should be omitted:

```
birthdate=mdy(birthmonth,birthday,birthyear;
```

Program 4.10: Estimation of Patient Age

```
/*1*/
data patient_healthcondition (drop=birthday birthmonth birthyear);
    set patient_healthcondition;

    Birthdate=mdy(birthmonth,birthDay,birthyear);
    format birthdate mmddyy10.;

    Age=(dateofonset - birthdate) / 365.2422;
    format age 6.1;

run;
```

4.6. Conversion of Variable Type to Numeric/Character

Sometimes you need to convert the variable type from character to numeric or from numeric to character. The PUT and INPUT functions can be utilized to convert a variable from numeric to character, or from character to numeric, respectively. By using these functions, you create a new variable with a new name. If you need the new variable to have the same original variable name, then you should drop the original variable and rename the new variable to the original name using RENAME function. In Example 1 of Program 4.11, first you create a temporary Exam data set from EHRDate.Exam table (optional), then you convert the Patient_ID, which is a numeric variable to a character variable (Char_var), then by dropping the old Patient_ID and renaming the Char_var to Patient_ID, you get a character type Patient_ID. In Example 2 of Program 4.11, you reverse the procedure by using the same method to convert the character Patient_ID to an integer. Conversion of character variables to numeric ones can also be carried out by adding "0" or by multiplying by 1 as neutral number to a character variable as you see in Example 3 of Program 4.11; however, this method is considered naïve method and should be avoided. Because we cannot tell the arithmetic operation what format should be applied to the number stored as text and sometimes the results are unpredictable.

Program 4.11: Conversion of Variable Type to Numeric/Character

```
/*Example 1*/
data exam (drop=patient_id);
      set ehrdata.exam;
      char_var=put(patient_id, 20.);
      rename char_var=patient_id;
run;

/* Example 2*/
data exam (drop=patient_id);
      set exam;
      numeric_var=input(patient_id, 20.);
      rename numeric_var=patient_id;
run;

/* Example 3*/
data exam (drop=patient_id);
      set exam;
      numeric_var=patient_id + 0;
      rename numeric_var=patient_id;
run;
```

4.7. Importance of Patient Encounter Date

The patient encounter date probably is the most important date in every EHR database. In most cases, the Encounter table that contains this date is a standalone table, and the encounter date does not have any relationship with other dates such as service date, date created, and so on. But what is the exact definition of encounter date? The fact is that there is no unique or standard definition for patient encounter date and that the recorded encounter dates depend on the definition of healthcare provider and encounter itself.

The definitions of "healthcare provider" and "encounter" are changeable from one organization to another one. Here, a definition from the United States Health Information Knowledgebase (2008) is demonstrated as an example. According to the definition, encounter date is the time of the patient presentation for care: arrival time (initial triage time) or the registration time for inpatients or check-in time for ambulatory settings.

It is important to remember that, for the purpose of analytical procedures, this definition and the dates that are provided by this definition, might not necessarily cover all interactions that patients have with healthcare providers, and consequently not adequate for statistical analysis. Accordingly, those research projects such as cross-sectional studies or disease case validations that depend on encounter date may suffer from incomprehensive encounter date. You may need to do some investigations to find out if the available encounter date is truly covering all patient interactions with providers or not, and if not, then you need to create a new encounter date that covers all possible encounters. *This new and inclusive encounter date can be used as a source **to indicate the existence of patients in the EHR database** during a certain period and to collect information from the patients between two cutoff dates and not just as a variable that covers some selected encounters.* Here is an example. Suppose for a cross-sectional study you need to collect patient information for those who have had encounter from January 1st, 2017, to January 1st, 2020, using the encounter dates available in the following records:

Patient	Encounter Date
A	14-07-2013
A	**25-11-2018**
A	05-03-2009
A	08-03-2009
B	**25-07-2017**
B	**23-07-2018**
B	27-06-2013
B	25-11-2016
C	.
C	.
C	.

According to the encounter date, only three records (in bold) must be considered for analysis: one record from patient A and two records from patient B. Thus, patient C will be dropped from further analysis.

However, after carefully investigating other tables, you may find the following records from the HealthCondition table for patient C:

Patient	DateOfOnset
C	21-09-2006
C	21-01-2018
C	14-06-2019

According to the HealthCondition table, there were at least two records in 2018 and 2019, which indicates that patient C in fact existed in your database and the onset of disease was between 2017 and 2020. This simple example shows you the consequence of using a defective encounter date and the possible bias that it may cause. You may notice that, in this example, patient C does not have records in the Encounter table, but there are cases where some patients may have records in the Encounter table, but the Encounter table does not show all their interactions with providers. To fix any of these problems, first you need to investigate the completeness of the Encounter table and then create a new encounter date that covers all possible interactions.

4.7.1. Investigation on the Completeness of Encounter Date

For simplicity, we focus here only on the records of those patients who are missing in the Encounter table, but they have records in other tables that are going to be discussed. The solution for fixing this problem can also be used to fix a defective encounter date that does not cover all possible patient interactions. You can easily investigate the completeness of the Encounter table using Program 4.12. In this program, first you sort and merge all EHR tables that have records of patient interaction with healthcare provider (except Encounter table), then you compare the created output data set and its encounter dates with those from the Encounter table. For this program, you should use the AC and A options of the match-merge program that you learned from Program 4.3 and Table 4.1. Finally, you can see the result of your investigation by printing some of the records. The created missing_in_encounter table contains all patients without any encounter date.

Program 4.12: Finding Patients without Encounter Date

```
proc sort data=ehrdata.allergy;
      by patient_id;

proc sort data=ehrdata.billing;
      by patient_id;

proc sort data=ehrdata.encounterdiagnosis;
      by patient_id;

proc sort data=ehrdata.exam;
      by patient_id;

proc sort data=ehrdata.healthcondition;
      by patient_id;

proc sort data=ehrdata.medication;
      by patient_id;

proc sort data=ehrdata.patient;
      by patient_id;

proc sort data=ehrdata.referral;
      by patient_id;

proc sort data=ehrdata.riskfactor;
      by patient_id;

proc sort data=ehrdata.vaccine;
      by patient_id;
run;

data all (keep=patient_id);
      merge ehrdata.patient(in=A) ehrdata.allergy (in=B) ehrdata.billing(in=C)
            ehrdata.encounterdiagnosis(in=D) ehrdata.exam(in=E)
            ehrdata.healthcondition(in=F)
      ehrdata.medication(in=G) ehrdata.referral(in=H)
            ehrdata.riskfactor(in=I)
      ehrdata.vaccine(in=J);
            by patient_id;

            if A=1 then
                  output all;
run;
```

```
proc sort data=ehrdata.encounter;
      by patient_id;
run;

data missing_in_encounter (keep=patient_id);
      merge all (in=A) ehrdata.encounter(in=B);
      by patient_id;

      if (A=1 and B=0) then
            output missing_in_encounter;
run;

proc print data=missing_in_encounter(obs=100);
run;
```

4.7.2. Making an Inclusive Encounter Date

All available and valid dates in different EHR data sets can be added to the current encounter date to make a new and inclusive encounter date. As mentioned earlier, the reason to make such a comprehensive date is for selection of the patient between two cutoff dates. Such an encounter date might not necessarily be equal with the medical definition or application for the encounter. Since the accuracy of different dates in EHR tables depends on the quality of data and subject to different criteria, it is worthwhile that before adding any date to the current encounter date, you consult with your data manager or administrator about the accuracy of each available date. For example, in a Billing table that contains both service date and date created, if the service date is more accurate than the date created, then the priority for adding these dates to your encounter date is with service date.

To add any dates to your current encounter date, first you need to change the name of date to encounter date, then you need to merge tables that contain those extra dates by Patient_ID. Program 4.13 shows you how you can add more dates from other EHRData tables to the Encounter table and create an inclusive encounter date. In the program, first a temporary data set is created from each EHR data set, then the most accurate date is selected and renamed using RENAME function. For example, from EHRData. Allergy table, StartDate is chosen and renamed to EncounterDate. Then the created data sets are sorted by Patient_ID. Both Encounter table and Patient Table are also sorted by their Patient_ID. Next, the created tables are merged with Encounter table and Patient table. The product of this match-merge (All_Encounter) contains all valid dates. At the end, since other variables such as Sex and BirthDay in the data set are consistent, duplicate observations with Patient_ID and EncounterDate are dropped from the data set.

Program 4.13: Making an Inclusive Encounter Date

```
data allergy (keep=patient_id StartDate);
    set ehrdata.allergy;

data allergy;
    set allergy;
    rename StartDate=encounterdate;

proc sort data=allergy;
    key patient_id/ ascending;
run;

data billing (keep=patient_id ServiceDate);
    set ehrdata.billing;

data billing;
    set billing;
    rename ServiceDate=encounterdate;

proc sort data=billing;
    key patient_id/ ascending;
run;

data encounterdiagnosis (keep=patient_id ServiceDate);
    set ehrdata.encounterdiagnosis;

data encounterdiagnosis;
    set encounterdiagnosis;
    rename ServiceDate=encounterdate;

proc sort data=encounterdiagnosis;
    key patient_id/ ascending;
run;

data exam (keep=patient_id PerformedDate);
    set ehrdata.exam;

data exam;
    set exam;
    rename PerformedDate=encounterdate;

proc sort data=exam;
```

```
              key patient_id/ ascending;
    run;

    data healthcondition (keep=patient_id DateOfOnset);
            set ehrdata.healthcondition;

    data healthcondition;
            set healthcondition;
            rename DateOfOnset=encounterdate;

    proc sort data=healthcondition;
            key patient_id/ ascending;
    run;
    data medication (keep=patient_id StartDate);
            set ehrdata.medication;
    data medication;
            set medication;
            rename StartDate=encounterdate;

    proc sort data=medication;
            key patient_id/ ascending;
    run;

    data referral (keep=patient_id DateCreated);
            set ehrdata.referral;

    data referral;
            set referral;
            rename DateCreated=encounterdate;

    proc sort data=referral;
            key patient_id/ ascending;
    run;

    data riskfactor (keep=patient_id PerformedDate);
            set ehrdata.riskfactor;

    data riskfactor;
            set riskfactor;
            rename PerformedDate=encounterdate;

    proc sort data=riskfactor;
            key patient_id/ ascending;
    run;

    data vaccine (keep=patient_id GivenDate);
            set ehrdata.vaccine;

    data vaccine;
```

```
        set vaccine;
        rename GivenDate=encounterdate;

proc sort data=vaccine;
        key patient_id/ ascending;
run;

data encounter (keep=patient_id EncounterDate);
        set ehrdata.encounter;

proc sort data=encounter;
        key patient_id/ ascending;
run;
data patient;
        set ehrdata.patient;

proc sort data=patient;
        key patient_id/ ascending;
run;

data all_encounter;
        merge patient(in=A) allergy (in=B) billing(in=C) encounterdiagnosis(in=D)
                exam(in=E) healthcondition(in=F) medication(in=G) referral(in=H)
                riskfactor(in=I) vaccine(in=J) encounter(in=K);
        by patient_id;

        if A=1 then
                output all_encounter;
run;

proc sort data=all_encounter nodupkey;
        by patient_id encounterdate;
run;
```

References

Foley M. J. MERGING vs. JOINING: Comparing the DATA Step with SQL. Available at: https://pdfs.semanticscholar.org/e21e/33fe735df1b6e14a6dacd77ac905e7d606eb.pdf.

Harris S. and Houser S. H. 2018. Double Trouble—Using Health Informatics to Tackle Duplicate Medical Record Issues. *Journal of AHIMA*. 89, no. 8: 20–23.

How to Read Two-Digit Years Using YEARCUTOFF=. Available at: https://v8doc.sas.com/sashtml/lrcon/z1330270.htm#z1300854.

United States Health Information Knowledgebase, 2008. Available at: https://ushik.ahrq.gov/ViewItemDetails?system=mdr&itemKey=84803000.

Part II: Analysis of Longitudinal EHR Data

Chapter 5

Data Extraction from Text and Analysis: Adverse Events Following Immunization

Abstract

There is a lot of useful healthcare information buried within provider description notes, requiring expensive and tedious manual chart review to identify, extract, and analyze. While there are some advanced text mining techniques for discovering and extracting information buried in unstructured data such as Natural Language Processing (NLP), the technical skills and software needed for such techniques are major barriers for medical researchers to implement these methods in their projects. In this chapter and the next chapters, a research question is submitted and a methodology for the step-by-step solution of the problem is proposed. The goal is for you to learn the SAS programming and statistical techniques by having hand-on experience.

5.1. Objectives

Immunization strategies have allowed important achievements in public health, such as the control or eradication of many communicable diseases. Despite these benefits, vaccines, like any other pharmaceutical product, may have risks, mostly associated with reactions. Although most reactions to vaccines are reported as discomfort, induration at the location of the immunization, and pain (Poland et al., 2009); nevertheless, concerns regarding the safety of vaccines have made countries create surveillance systems to monitor adverse reactions. One of these surveillance systems is the Vaccine Adverse Event Reporting System (VAERS), which makes its data publicly available in CSV format from the U.S. Department of Health and Human Services (HHS)[1].

---

[1] http://vaers.hhs.gov.

For this chapter, you are going to use some simple programming techniques to carry out the basic tasks such as extraction of information from unstructured data, conversion of text to numeric variables, and eventually analyzing data. The data set EHRData.Vaers contains unstructured information about the adverse reactions following immunization that are reported by vaccine manufacturers and health care providers. The EHRData.Vaers data set was created from vaersdata and vaersvax of the VAERS database. The objectives of this descriptive and analytical study are to do the following:

1. Analyze the frequency and distribution of the most common adverse effects of vaccination.
2. Investigate the risks of adverse effects related to the age and sex of the vaccine receiver.

5.2. Methodology

5.2.1. Changing Lower Case to Upper Case and Vice Versa

Character variables in the EHRData.Vaers data set contain a mix of uppercase and lowercase text. Although in SAS some names such as library, file, and variable names are not case-sensitive, the operations on string variables are case-sensitive. Thus, when you need to make string operations or execute character values through SAS logical statements, texts with both uppercase and lowercase may not be used properly, and you may need to take some precautions. To avoid the problems associated with case sensitivity, you should either convert texts to uppercase or lowercase. You can use the first part of Program 5.1 to convert the contents of all character variables to uppercase. To change all contents of character variables to lowercase, you just need to replace the UPCASE statement with LOWCASE in the same program. If you only need to change the contents of one variable, you can do so by using the second part of the program. In the second part, only the content of Symptom_text variable is converted to uppercase.

Program 5.1: Changing Character Variable Data from Lowercase to Uppercase or Vice Versa

```
/*Part 1*/
```

Data Extraction from Text and Analysis

```
data ehrdata.vaers;
    set ehrdata.vaers;
    array chars[*] _character_;

    do i=1 to dim(chars);
        chars[i]=upcase(chars[i]);
    end;
    drop i;
run;

/*Part 2*/
data ehrdata.vaers;
    set ehrdata.vaers;
    symptom_text=upcase(symptom_text);
run;
```

5.2.2. Parsing the Character String

Use unstructured information from the Symptom_text of EHRData.Vaers to extract useful information including adverse effects of vaccines. Some of the most frequent adverse effects are RASH, CHILLS, ERYTHEMA including INJECTION SITE ERYTHEMA, PYREXIA (FEVER), ARTHRALGIA (PAIN IN JOINT), ASTHENIA (including WEAKNESS, FATIGUE or TIREDNESS), and NAUSEA. These symptoms need to be extracted from the text and converted to dummy variables for further analysis. Program 5.2 shows you step by step to create a new data set by converting the text to these variables.

5.2.2.1. Step 1

First you create a data set from ehrdata.vaers for each adverse effect (Vaers1,...) by keeping only those variables that are needed for analysis.

Dealing with negative statements in a text (negation), is perhaps the most problematic issue with unstructured data. Words such as "no", "never", and so on when attended with target words, they can contradict or deny the target word. Sometimes the phrases with negation are difficult to identify or convert appropriately. Look at the following examples from Symptom_text.

- Example 1:
  - *"pt came to the clinic on 2/11/2020 c/o hives to left arm. stated it started on 02/10/2020. no pain, no fever, **NO CHILLS**. just*

very itchy. given a dose of cetirizine 10 mg and applied hydrocortisone."

In this example, although there is a "CHILLS" in patient's statement, it is accompanied with "NO." Therefore, this case cannot be considered as a positive case of "Chills" symptom. Now, look at the second example, which is more complex.

- Example 2:
  - *"injection very painful originally, pain at site becoming more severe over course of day, by 3:30 pm pain unbearable, felt like I ran into a brick wall, unable to lift my left arm, had to support it at elbow with right hand. thick swelling at injection site, **CHILLS** and fever from 100 degrees to 101 degrees. i was in bed by 7:30 pm, fitful sleep for most of night. by 6:00 am next morning, **NO CHILLS**, no fever, soreness still in arm, but no longer extreme pain. soreness lasted for another day or two."*

In the second example, there are two cases of "**CHILLS.**" Here, a positive case of "**CHILLS**" followed by a "**NO CHILLS**" later, indicating the patient had chills symptoms before and later he/she became better. Therefore, this patient should be counted as positive case for "Chills."

The question is, how you can convert the first case to "1" for Chills and "0" for the second case? While there might be different techniques to do this task, one simple method is just substituting the word(s) containing both the target (e.g., **CHILLS**) and negative word to something neutral first (e.g., XXXX) and then converting the target name that is left in the text to numeric variable.

The TRANWRD (translate word) function can be used to perform a search and replace operation on a string variable (Cody 2005). In the step 1 of Program 5.2, you substitute the negations with XXXX, assuming that "No" is the only word that is used for negations. Then, using the FIND function, you search the entire Symptom_text for the key words of adverse effects and if the program finds those key words, it will put 1 for the presence of the key words and 0 otherwise.

Table 5.1. The first five rows of the most frequent adverse effects of vaccination

Obs	Vaers_id	State	Age	Sex	Rash	Chills	Erythema	Pyrexia	Arthralgia	Asthenia	Nausea
1	855017	HI	55	F	0	1	0	1	0	0	0
2	855018	WI	68	F	0	1	0	1	0	1	0
3	855019		50	F	1	0	0	0	0	0	0
4	855020	TX	67	F	0	1	0	1	1	0	0
5	855021		73	F	1	1	0	0	0	0	1

5.2.2.2. Step 2

Next, you remove duplicate data from each Vaers_ID (vaccine receiver) by sorting the data set in a DESCENDING order and using NODUPKEY statements. Consequently, if duplicate observations contain both 0 and 1, only 1 will remain in the data set. When there are several variables in a data set and you need to remove duplicate observations for all variables, the process of removing duplicate data should be carried out by creating a new temporary data set for each variable then after removing duplicate data for each data set, the data sets can be merged to create a new data set containing all variables. Otherwise, if you try to remove duplicate data for all variables at the same time in a data set and in one single step, you may see unpredictable results.

Program 5.2: Conversion of Text from Adverse Effects of Vaccination to Numeric Variables

```
/*Step 1*/
data vaers(keep=vaers_id state age sex vax_type
symptom_text);
     set ehrdata.vaers;

data vaers;
     set vaers;
     symptom_text=tranwrd(symptom_text, 'NO RASH',
'XXXX');
     symptom_text=tranwrd(symptom_text, 'NO CHILLS',
'XXXX');
     symptom_text=tranwrd(symptom_text, 'NO ERYTHEMA',
'XXXX');
     symptom_text=tranwrd(symptom_text, 'NO INJECTION SITE
ERYTHEMA', 'XXXX');
     symptom_text=tranwrd(symptom_text, 'NO PYREXIA',
'XXXX');
     symptom_text=tranwrd(symptom_text, 'NO FEVER',
'XXXX');
     symptom_text=tranwrd(symptom_text, 'NO ARTHRALGIA',
'XXXX');
     symptom_text=tranwrd(symptom_text, 'NO PAIN IN
JOINT', 'XXXX');
     symptom_text=tranwrd(symptom_text, 'NO JOINT PAIN',
'XXXX');
     symptom_text=tranwrd(symptom_text, 'NO ASTHENIA',
'XXXX');
     symptom_text=tranwrd(symptom_text, 'NO WEAKNESS',
'XXXX');
```

```
    symptom_text=tranwrd(symptom_text, 'NO FATIGUE',
'XXXX');
    symptom_text=tranwrd(symptom_text, 'NO TIREDNESS',
'XXXX');
    symptom_text=tranwrd(symptom_text, 'NO NAUSEA',
'XXXX');

      if find (symptom_text, 'RASH')then
            rash=1;
      else
            rash=0;

      if find (symptom_text, 'CHILLS')then
            chills=1;
      else
            chills=0;

      if find (symptom_text, 'ERYTHEMA') or find
(symptom_text,
            'INJECTION SITE ERYTHEMA')then
                  erythema=1;
      else
            erythema=0;

      if find (symptom_text, 'PYREXIA') or find
(symptom_text, 'FEVER')then
            pyrexia=1;
      else
            pyrexia=0;

      if find (symptom_text, 'ARTHRALGIA') or find
(symptom_text, 'PAIN IN JOINT')
            or find (symptom_text, 'JOINT PAIN') then
                  arthralgia=1;
      else
            arthralgia=0;

      if find (symptom_text, 'ASTHENIA') or find
(symptom_text, 'WEAKNESS') or
            find (symptom_text, 'FATIGUE') or find
(symptom_text, 'TIREDNESS')then
                  asthenia=1;
      else
            asthenia=0;

      if find (symptom_text, 'NAUSEA')then
            nausea=1;
      else
            nausea=0;
```

```
run;

data vaers(drop=symptom_text);
    set vaers;
run;

/*Step 2*/
data patients (keep=vaers_id state age sex);
    set vaers;

proc sort data=patients nodupkey;
    key vaers_id /ascending;
run;
data rash (keep=vaers_id rash);
    set vaers;

proc sort data=rash nodupkey;
    key vaers_id /ascending;
    key rash/descending;
run;

data chills (keep=vaers_id chills);
    set vaers;

proc sort data=chills nodupkey;
    key vaers_id /ascending;
    key chills/descending;
run;

data erythema (keep=vaers_id erythema);
    set vaers;

proc sort data=erythema nodupkey;
    key vaers_id /ascending;
    key erythema /descending;
run;

data pyrexia (keep=vaers_id pyrexia);
    set vaers;

proc sort data=pyrexia nodupkey;
    key vaers_id /ascending;
    key pyrexia/descending;
run;

data arthralgia (keep=vaers_id arthralgia);
    set vaers;

proc sort data=arthralgia nodupkey;
```

```
            key vaers_id /ascending;
            key arthralgia/descending;
    run;

    data asthenia (keep=vaers_id asthenia);
            set vaers;

    proc sort data=asthenia nodupkey;
            key vaers_id /ascending;
            key asthenia/descending;
    run;

    data nausea (keep=vaers_id nausea);
            set vaers;

    proc sort data=nausea nodupkey;
            key vaers_id /ascending;
            key nausea/descending;
    run;

    data ehrdata.vaers1;
            merge patients(in=A) rash(in=B) chills (in=C)
    erythema(in=D) pyrexia(in=E)
                    arthralgia(in=F) asthenia(in=G) nausea(in=H);
            by vaers_id;

            if A=1 then
                    output ehrdata.vaers1;
    run;
```

The final product of Program 5.2 (EHRData.vaers1) is a data set containing all receivers of vaccines with adverse effects in separate columns and with only one single observation (row) for each receiver. Table 5.1 illustrates the first five observations of the data set.

5.3. Analysis and Results

Now is the time to perform analysis for each objective.

Objective 1: Analyze the frequency and distribution of the most common adverse effects of vaccination.

Using PROC FREQ, you can easily calculate the frequency of each adverse effect. Part 1 and part 2 of Program 5.3 show you how you can achieve this goal. In part 1, the frequency of each adverse effect is estimated.

For example, according to the results of this part of analysis, 6.75% of vaccine receivers reported a *side effect* with the rash symptom (Table 5.2).

Program 5.3: Frequency and Distribution of the Most Common Adverse Effects of Vaccination

```
/*Part 1*/
proc freq data=ehrdata.vaers1 order=freq;
        tables rash chills erythema pyrexia arthralgia
asthenia nausea / norow nocol
                nocum;
run;

/*Part 2*/
proc freq data=ehrdata.vaers1 order=freq;
        tables
rash*chills*erythema*pyrexia*arthralgia*asthenia*nausea /
list norow
                nocol nocum;
run;
```

Table 5.2. Frequency of patients with and without "rash" symptom following vaccination

Rash	Frequency	Percent
0	10631	90.79
1	1079	9.21

In Part 2 of the same program, the frequency of all combinations **of the side effects** is calculated. The first five combinations of the **side effects** are shown in Table 5.3. For example, according to this table, 66.13% of the receiver did not report any of those adverse effects and 0.44% of patients showed both asthenia and Nausea and so on.

Table 5.3. The first five combinations of adverse effects of vaccines

Rash	Chills	Erythema	Pyrexia	Arthralgia	Asthenia	Nausea	Frequency	Percent
0	0	0	0	0	0	0	7744	66.13
0	0	0	0	0	0	1	237	2.02
0	0	0	0	0	1	0	348	2.97
0	0	0	0	0	1	1	51	0.44
0	0	0	0	1	0	0	56	0.48

Objective 2: Investigate the risk of adverse effects related to the age and sex of the vaccine receiver.

The aim of this part of study is to investigate the age- and sex-specific incidence rates of suspected adverse vaccination reactions recorded by practitioners. The relative risk and 95% confidence intervals of having an adverse reaction recorded by practitioners for females compared with males (reference group) in each of the age groups is calculated. You also calculate the relative risk and 95% confidence limits of having an adverse event recorded by practitioners in each age group using the < 20-**year** age band as the reference group.

In Part 1 of Program 5.4, first you sort data by age, then using PROC FORMAT you implement the age category. Next, using PROC FREQ you calculate the frequency of each symptom based on age and sex. Tables 5.4 and 5.5 reveal the frequency of developing a rash after vaccination by sex and age, respectively.

In Part 2, using PROC GENMOD you estimate and compare the risk of having a rash after vaccination for different age and sex categories. In PROC GENMOD, all categorical variables (sex and age) that are part of model must be mentioned in CLASS statement. The REF="M" and REF="A: < 20" statements requests SAS to use Male and Age category A: < 20 as references for risk comparisons. The PARAM=GLM specifies the GLM parameterization method for the classification variables. This model also specifies DIST = BIN to indicate that you are interested in a binomial distribution with LINK = LOGIT for the logit function. The relative risk or the risk ratio of getting a rash after vaccination and its confidence intervals can be estimated using LSMEANS statement in the model.

According to the results and the Parameter Estimates table, the linear effect of the predictors is not significant. Although the results are not significant, for the purpose of this tutorial, let us continue and see how the relative risk can be interpreted. The result from the Least Squares Means tables provides estimates of the log relative risk (Estimate) and relative risk (Exponentiated) estimates. In this example, the relative risk event of having a rash after vaccination for female receivers is 0.6 (95% CL: 0.2-1.9) compared to male receivers (Table 5.6). Since, the risk ratio is less than 1, this suggests a reduced risk in the female group.

Program 5.4: The Risk of Adverse Effects Related to the Age and Sex of the Vaccine Recipient

```
/*Part 1*/
proc sort data=ehrdata.vaers1 nodupkey;
        key age/ascending;
run;

proc format;
        value agefmt 0 - <20='A: < 20' 20 - <40='B: 20 to 39'
40 - <60='C: 40 to 59'
                60 - high='D: 60+';
run;

proc freq data=ehrdata.vaers1;
        tables age*(rash chills erythema pyrexia arthralgia
asthenia) / norow nocol
                nocum;
        format age agefmt.;
run;

proc freq data=ehrdata.vaers1 order=freq;
        tables sex*(rash chills erythema pyrexia arthralgia
asthenia) / norow nocol
                nocum;
run;

/*Part 2*/
proc genmod data=ehrdata.vaers1 descending;
        class sex (ref="M") age(ref="A: < 20")/ param=glm;
        model rash=sex age / dist=bin link=logit;
        lsmeans age / diff=control("A: < 20")exp cl;
        lsmeans sex / diff=control("M") exp cl;
        format age agefmt.;
run;
```

According to VAERS, the vaccine adverse event reports alone cannot be used to determine if a vaccine caused or contributed to an adverse event or illness. Because the reports are voluntary, they are subject to biases and may contain information that is incomplete or inaccurate. This creates specific limitations on how the results should be used scientifically. Therefore, the results and findings of this chapter should be interpreted with these limitations in mind and the results should only be considered for the purpose of the statistical/programming study and not as evidence for or against a specified vaccine.

Table 5.4. The frequency and percentage of developing a rash following vaccine by sex (M=Male, F=Female, U=Blank)

Sex	Chills		Total
	0	1	
F	5751	639	6390
	49.11	5.46	54.57
M	3042	360	3402
	25.98	3.07	29.05
U	1838	80	1918
	15.7	0.68	16.38
Total	10631	1079	11710
	90.79	9.21	100

Table 5.5. The frequency and percentage of developing a rash following vaccine by age

Age	Chills		Total
	0	1	
A: <20	2007	245	2252
	26.23	3.2	29.43
B: 20 to 39	690	72	762
	9.02	0.94	9.96
C: 40 to 59	1293	167	1460
	16.9	2.18	19.08
D: 60+	2786	391	3177
	36.41	5.11	41.52
Total	6776	875	7651
	88.56	11.44	100

Table 5.6. The relative risk of developing a rash after vaccination by sex (M=Male, F=Female, U=Unknown)

Sex	Sex	Estimate	Standard Error	z Value	Pr > |z|	Alpha	Lower	Upper	Exponentiated	Exponentiated Lower	Exponentiated Upper
F	M	-0.5	0.6	-0.9	0.4	0.1	-1.6	0.6	0.6	0.2	1.9
U	M	-24.0	111554.0	0.0	1.0	0.1	-218666.0	218618.0	0.0	0	Infty

References

Cody R., *An Introduction to SAS® Character Functions* (Including Some New SAS®9 Functions). 2005. Available at: https://support.sas.com/resources/papers/proceedings/proceedings/sugi30/233-30.pdf.

Poland GA, Ovsyannikova IG, Jacobson RM. Adversomics: The emerging field of vaccine adverse event immunogenetics. *Pediatr. Infect. Dis. J.* 2009, 28, 431–432.

Chapter 6

Prevalence Estimation for Acute Diseases (A Cross-Sectional Cohort Study)

Abstract

In epidemiology, the cross-sectional cohort design is utilized for sampling from population in a cross-sectional fashion (over a specified period) to create a cohort with patients and then retrospectively investigate the history of exposures and outcomes in the members of that cohort. The study cohort has been defined as the set of all individuals from a given source population who are available for evaluation at a specific calendar time point, T1 (Hudson et al., 2005). Usually, T1 will be the present, but it can be considered as past too. To extract patient information from EHR data and estimate prevalence or other statistics using cross-sectional cohort study, one needs to look patient records retrospectively (looking backward) because the available data reflect only information from the past. Suppose in Figure 6.1 that the arrow represents the stream of the EHR data, and each circle indicates a patient. Also suppose that it is the year 2020 and you are interested in creating a cohort population from 2015 to 2017 to investigate their information. This is going to be a retrospective cross-sectional cohort study of a two-year contact group with four patients regardless of their disease conditions (with or without disease, white circles).

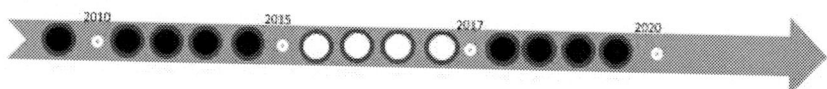

Figure 6.1. Retrospective cross-sectional cohort study with four patients (white circles) from 2015–2017.

6.1. Objectives

This chapter aims to help you with extraction and analyzing records between two time periods for acute (non-chronic) diseases. For this chapter you are going to estimate crude, and sex-age adjusted (standardized) prevalence of herpes Zoster (HZ) disease including HZ-related nervous system complication as an example of acute diseases using a two-year contact group (2018–2020) of patients from EHRData. Here defining the study population as a two-year contact group is arbitrary and it can be defined as n-year contact group. The objectives of this study are the following:

1. Estimate the descriptive statistics for population, total crude prevalence for HZ with 95% confidence interval and prevalence by age and sex and the corresponding odds ratio for patients >18 years of age who had at least one visit with their primary health care provider within 2018-2020.
2. Estimate the sex-age adjusted prevalence of HZ for the same population.

6.2. Methodology

6.2.1. Case Definition

A case definition based on rule-based system for HZ using ICD-9 codes (053 or 053.**) was previously reported by Queenan et al. (2017). Based on the definition, the diagnosis of HZ with or without related Nervous System Complication includes patients who have an infection with HZ, Varicella-HZ virus infection, shingles and/or have been diagnosed with any nervous system complication. It does not include chicken pox, genital herpes, or herpes simplex labialis. Using ICD-10 codes as suggested by Kim et al. (2018) for HZ, B02* codes can be used to extract HZ cases. For patients with HZ cases with or without nervous system complication, any occurrence of the ICD-10 B02 and sub codes (B02*) in Billing, Encounter_Diagnosis, and Health_Condition can be utilized to extract HZ cases.

6.2.2. Crude Prevalence Estimation

Perhaps the best way to start programming for research projects that involve prevalence or incidence estimation for acute (non-chronic) diseases using EHR data is creating a cohort data set containing all patients for the fraction of the time that you need for analysis. The total number of patients in the cohort data set will be the denominator of the following prevalence equation:

$$\text{Prevalence} = \frac{\text{Number of cases in the sample}}{\text{Total number of patients}} \quad (1)$$

Hence, for this study the denominator of the prevalence equation is all patients who have at least one interaction or visit with healthcare provider between 2018 and 2020 (two-year contact group). The numerator is the total number of patients who were diagnosed with HZ during that period. This prevalence is also called *period prevalence*, which is different from *point prevalence* and *lifetime prevalence*. The point prevalence is the proportion of a population that has the characteristic at a specific point in time, and the lifetime prevalence is the proportion of a population who, in their lifetime (or in the entire database) has ever had the characteristic.

Prevalence may be reported as a percentage or as the number of cases per 10,000 or 100,000 people. Thus, to calculate the prevalence of HZ as percentage, the following equation can be used:

$$\text{Prevalence of HZ} = \left(\frac{\text{Number of cases with HZ in 2018-2020}}{\text{Total number of patients in 2018-2020}} \right) \times 100 \quad (2)$$

6.2.3. Age-Sex Adjustment (Standardization)

Crude rates of a disease can be influenced by both age and sex. The age and sex distributions of two populations can be different and even for the same population they can change over time. Age-sex adjustment ensures that differences in prevalence of a disease from one year to another, or from one location to another or between two populations, are not because of differences in the age-sex distribution of the populations being compared. The terms "adjustment" and "standardization" refer to procedures for facilitating the comparison of summary measures across groups. Adjustment, the more general term, involves both standardization and other techniques for eliminating the effects of elements that alter or confound a comparison. Standardization refers to methods of adjustment based on weighted averages (Schoenbach, 1999) using a reference population. Standardization can be done by direct or indirect methods (Yuan, 2013). For direct standardization, you will use the weights from a reference population to compute the weighted average of stratum-specific rate or risk estimates in the study population. For indirect standardization you will use the stratum-specific rate or risk estimates in the reference population to compute the expected number of events in the study population.

Sex-age standardized total and stratified (within classes) prevalence estimation using direct or indirect methods for a single population, and a reference population can be done by both PROC STDRATE and spreadsheet software such as Excel (Bains, 2009). Remember, in SAS, PROC STDRATE can be used to obtain sex-age standardized **total** prevalence for a **single** population or sex-age standardized **total** and **stratified** prevalence for **two** sample populations using a reference population. In this chapter, since you are dealing with a **single** population, to obtain sex-age stratified prevalence standardization using PROC STDRATE, you need to do some tricks or conversely you can use Excel software.

6.3. Analysis and Results

6.3.1. Objective 1: Crude Prevalence Estimation

The following step-by-step guideline directs you toward successful statistical programming:

1. Sort both the Patient and Encounter tables first, merge them, then create a subset of data for those patients that had at least one visit with the primary care provider between Jan. 1st 2018 to Dec. 31st 2020. Such a subset of data is your two-year contact group (denominator) for the equation (2).
2. Merge the product of step 1 with the tables that contain useful information for the case definition in Section 6.2.1. Such information for this study can be derived from Billing, Encounter_Diagnosis, and Health_Condition tables.
3. Create a new variable (HZ) for the presence or absence of HZ disease by converting ICD-10 (B02*) codes to dummy variables. Calculate patient age for the onset of HZ using OnsetDate in HealthCondition table and subset data by removing those who are younger than 18 years old at the time of the onset of zoster.
4. Sort data for HZ variable in a descending order, then remove duplicate observations.

5. Estimate total crude prevalence, prevalence by age and sex, and odds ratio.
6. Estimate the sex-age standardized prevalence.

Objective 1: Estimate the descriptive statistics for population, unadjusted prevalence with 95% confidence interval, and prevalence by age and sex and the corresponding odds ratio for patients >18 years of age who had at least one visit with their primary health care provider within 2018-2020.

6.3.1.1. Step 1

As mentioned earlier, you need to make a subset of data from patients who had at least one visit with their primary care provider between Jan. 1st 2018 to Dec. 31st 2020. Such a population can be derived from the Patient table, but since this table does not cover all encounter dates, you need to merge this table with the Encounter table. Remember, if you have a reason to believe that the Encounter table also does not cover all encounter dates, then you need to create a new encounter date that can cover all patient encounters by merging all EHR tables and using their available valid dates. For this exercise, suppose that the Encounter date from the Encounter table is a comprehensive and sufficient date that covers all possible encounter dates. The match-merge technique, which was discussed in Chapter 4, can be used to create the cohort data set for further steps. You can use Program 6.1 to carry out the first step.

Program 6.1: Creating Subset Data (Denominator) Using Match-Merge Technique

```
proc sort data=ehrdata.patient;
     by patient_id;
run;

proc sort data=ehrdata.encounter;
     by patient_id;
run;

data patient_encounter (keep=patient_id sex birthday
birthmonth birthyear
             encounterdate);
     format EncounterDate mmddyy10.;
     merge ehrdata.patient (in=A) ehrdata.encounter
(in=B);
```

```
                by patient_id;

                if (A=1 or B=1) then
                        output patient_encounter;
run;

data patient_encounter;
        set patient_encounter;

                if '1jan2018'd <=encounterdate <='31dec2020'd;
run;
```

In Program 6.1, data from both the Patient and Encounter tables are sorted by Patient_ID first, then they are merged, and the subset data is created using two cut-off dates.

6.3.1.2. Step 2

For this step, you need to merge the product of Step 1 which is Patient_encounter data set with Billing, Encounter_Diagnosis and Health_Condition tables. Program 6.2 can be used for this part of analysis.

Program 6.2: Adding Billing, Encounter_Diagnosis and Health_Condition Data to Patient_encounter Data Set

```
proc sort data=ehrdata.billing;
        by patient_id;
run;

proc sort data=ehrdata.encounterdiagnosis;
        by patient_id;
run;

proc sort data=ehrdata.healthcondition;
        by patient_id;
run;

data ehrdata.HZ (keep=patient_id sex birthday birthmonth birthyear
                    encounterdate diagnosiscode_calc dateofonset);
        format encounterdate mmddyy10.;
        merge patient_encounter (in=A) ehrdata.billing (in=B)
                ehrdata.encounterdiagnosis (in=C)
ehrdata.healthcondition (in=D);
        by patient_id;
```

```
        if (A=1) then
                output ehrdata.HZ;
run;
```

6.3.1.3. Step 3

For this step, you will create a new dummy variable (HZ) by converting all ICD-10 codes that start with B02 and later by writing a program you will calculate patient age at the onset of HZ diagnosis using OnsetDate variable (Program 6.3). Next, you will remove all unnecessary variables and limit your analysis to those patients older than 18.

Program 6.3: Creating a HZ Variable and Estimation of Patient Age at Onset of the Disease

```
data ehrdata.HZ;
        set ehrdata.HZ;

        if (substr(diagnosiscode_calc, 1, 3))="B02" then
                HZ=1;
        else
                HZ=0;
        birthdate=mdy(birthmonth, birthday, birthyear);
        format birthdate mmddyy10.;
        idate=(dateofonset);
        bdate=(birthdate);
        ageint=idate-bdate;
        age=ageint/365.2422;
        format age 6.1;
run;

data ehrdata.HZ (drop=encounterdate birthday birthmonth birthyear
                diagnosiscode_calc dateofonset birthdate idate bdate ageint);
        set ehrdata.HZ;
        where age>18;
run;
```

6.3.1.4. Step 4

By sorting HZ variable in a descending order and removing duplicate observations, the data set will be ready for prevalence estimation (Program 6.4).

Program 6.4: Removing Duplicate HZ Observations for Each Patient

```
proc sort data=ehrdata.HZ;
        key patient_id / ascending;
        key HZ / descending;
run;

data ehrdata.HZ;
        set ehrdata.HZ;
        by patient_id;

        if first.patient_id;
run;
```

6.3.1.5. Step 5

Using Program 6.5 you can estimate the descriptive statistics of age by sex for patients with or without the disease, the prevalence of HZ by age and gender, and the corresponding odds ratio in patients with at least one encounter over two years.

Program 6.5: Descriptive Statistics and Prevalence Estimation for HZ by Sex and Age

```
/*Section 1*/
proc format;
        value agefmt 20 - <40='A: < 40' 40 - <60='B: 40 to
60' 60 - high='C: 60+';
run;

/*Section 2*/
proc means data=ehrdata.HZ maxdec=1 mean clm range std;
        class sex;
        var age;
        where HZ=1;
title "age characteristics of patients with zoster";
run;

proc means data=ehrdata.HZ maxdec=1 mean clm range std;
        class sex;
        var age;
        where HZ=0;
title "age characteristics of patients without zoster";
run;

/*Section 3*/
proc means data=ehrdata.HZ maxdec=3 mean clm;
```

```
        var HZ;
run;

proc means data=ehrdata.HZ maxdec=3 mean clm;
        class age sex;
        var HZ;
        format age agefmt.;
run;

/*Section 4*/
proc genmod data=ehrdata.HZ descending;
        class sex (ref="Male") age(ref="A: < 40")/ param=glm;
        model HZ=sex age / dist=bin link=logit;
        lsmeans age / diff=control("A: < 40")exp cl;
        lsmeans sex / diff=control("Male") exp cl;
        lsmestimate sex 'Male vs Female' 1 -1 / exp cl;
        format age agefmt.;
run;
```

In the first section of Program 6.5, first you introduce the age category to SAS by using PROC FORMAT. Then in the second section, you estimate several statistics including mean, confidence limits, range, and standard deviations of patients age with or without HZ. In the third section, you will estimate the total prevalence of HZ and its 95% confidence interval and the prevalence by gender and age. By multiplying the prevalence and its confidence limits in 100, you can get prevalence as percentage. This can also be done by making a new variable using HZ variable that is multiplied in 100 and adding the formula into data step of the program, for example:

HZ100=HZ*100;

In the fourth section, you estimate odds ratios for age and sex using PROC GENMOD. When creating a logistic regression model by PROC GENMOD, you can use the EXP option together with an ESTIMATE, LSMEANS, or LSMESTIMATE statement to obtain an odds ratio estimate and corresponding confidence intervals. To use the LSMEANS or LSMESTIMATE statement, you must use the default parameterization (PARAM=GLM) in the CLASS statement. If you want to use an ESTIMATE statement to obtain an odds ratio, then you need to specify the contrast coefficients of a linear combination of model parameters, which is more complex than other statements. If you only need to compare the main effects and not interactions, then the LSMEANS statement may be the easiest method to do so. Adding the EXP option will exponentiate the log odds ratios, which will give you the odds ratio estimates.

Table 6.1 reveals age characteristics for patients with or without HZ. According to this table, the average age for female patients with HZ is 44.6 and for male patients is 57.1 years old. The age difference between the male and female is negligible for those without HZ.

Table 6.1. Age characteristics for patients with or without HZ

Sex	N	Mean	Lower 95% CL for Mean	Upper 95% CL for Mean	Range	Std Dev
With HZ						
Female	12	44.6	39.1	50.2	29.8	8.8
Male	4	57.1	50.5	63.7	9.4	4.2
Without HZ						
Female	303	45.4	44.2	46.6	51.1	10.6
Male	272	45.5	44.3	46.8	51.3	10.4

Table 6.2. Unadjusted (crude) prevalence of HZ by age and gender in patients with at least one encounter over two years

Age	Sex	N Obs	Prevalence (%)	Lower 95% CL for Mean	Upper 95% CL for Mean
A: < 40	Female	100	3.0	0	6.4
	Male	81	0	.	.
B: 40 to 60	Female	187	4.8	1.7	7.9
	Male	171	1.8	0	3.7
C: 60+	Female	28	0	.	.
	Male	24	4.2	0	12.8

According to the third section of Program 6.5, the overall crude prevalence of HZ for those over 18 years old and with at least one encounter over 2 years is 2.7% (95% CI: 1.4, 4.0). Table 6.2 presents the age and sex stratified prevalence of HZ in the EHRData. The prevalence increases by age in male patients. The prevalence of HZ is the highest amongst females in 40 to 60 age group. The lower bounds of confidence intervals with negative signs resulted from this part of analysis can be replaced with zero as the rates cannot be negative. Replacing negative numbers does not decrease the confidence level. The groups whose confidence interval includes a value of zero are considered as non-significant.

The result from the Least Squares Means tables provides estimates of the Odds ratio (**Exponentiated**) estimates (Table 6.3). Comparing the odds ratio, a female patient is 2.7 (95% CL: 0.9-8.6) times more likely to develop HZ compared to a male patient. Patients with age category B and C are 2.1 (95% CL: 0.6-7.6) and 1.2 (95% CL: 0.1-11.6) times more likely to develop HZ compared to A (Table 6.3). Here the significance level is 0.05 and the corresponding confidence level is 95%. In epidemiology, the null value for both relative risk and odds ratio is considered 1. If the 95% confidence interval does not include the null value, the finding is statistically significant. Here, the lower bounds of confidence intervals are less than 1 for odds ratio and the confidence interval includes the null value. Therefore, all effects of HZ for odds ratio are non-significant. These estimates are associated with wide confidence intervals because of the small number of patients with HZ, therefore the statistical power to detect a difference was small.

Table 6.3. Odds ratio and 95% confidence interval for HZ patients by gender and age

Effect	Label	Odds Ratio (Exponentiated)	Lower 95% CL for Odds Ratio (Exponentiated)	Upper 95% CL for Odds Ratio (Exponentiated)
Sex	Male vs Female	2.7	0.9	8.6
Age	A vs B	2.1	0.6	7.6
	A vs C	1.2	0.1	11.6

Objective 2: Estimate the sex-age adjusted prevalence of HZ for the same population.

6.3.2. Objective 2: Age-Sex Standardization

As you noticed from the results of Objective 1, crude prevalence of HZ can be influenced by both age and sex. To adjust for age-sex, a reference population is needed. Table 6.4 shows the annual estimates of the resident population for select age-sex groups in the United States in 2019 (U.S. Census Bureau, Population Division, 2020).

Obviously, the age-sex category (strata) of this table is not what you can use to adjust the prevalence, as the classes are different from the one that you used for crude prevalence estimation (Table 6.2). However, you can easily change it to something like Table 6.5 using Excel or any other spreadsheet software.

Using Program 6.6 you can estimate the total sex-age standardized prevalence of HZ. In the first section of this program, first you make EHRData.HZ ready for PROC FREQ by sorting data. Next, the FREQ procedure gives you the number of patients with HZ for each sex-age group. In the second section, you create a temporary data set (HZ) by information that you obtained from the previous step. The PYear variable is the total number of patients in each sex-age group. Like the second section, in the third section you will create another temporary data set (US) from Table 6.5. Again, the PYear in the US data set is the total number of populations for each group. In the fourth section, you will estimate the standardized total prevalence of HZ and its 95% confidence intervals.

Table 6.4. Annual estimates of the resident population for selected age-sex groups in the United States in 2019

Age	Male	Female
Under 5 years	10,009,207	9,567,476
5 to 9 years	10,322,762	9,873,133
10 to 14 years	10,618,261	10,180,007
15 to 19 years	10,745,607	10,308,963
20 to 24 years	11,064,752	10,568,188
25 to 29 years	12,004,570	11,504,446
30 to 34 years	11,354,610	11,076,695
35 to 39 years	10,884,941	10,852,580
40 to 44 years	9,907,139	10,014,484
45 to 49 years	10,085,355	10,312,396
50 to 54 years	10,086,611	10,390,540
55 to 59 years	10,642,489	11,234,902
60 to 64 years	9,856,730	10,714,416
65 to 69 years	8,199,773	9,255,228
70 to 74 years	6,499,806	7,528,626
75 to 79 years	4,318,499	5,334,166
80 to 84 years	2,679,724	3,637,483
85 years and over	2,376,488	4,228,470
Total	161,657,324	166,582,199

Table 6.5. Annual estimates of the resident population for select age groups by sex for US in 2019

Age Category	Male	Female
20 - <40	45,308,873	44,001,909
40 - <60	40,721,594	41,952,322
60 - high	33,931,020	40,698,389

Table 6.6. Estimation of standardized prevalence of HZ by age and gender in patients with at least one encounter over two years using any spreadsheet software

Sex	Age	Study Population		Standard Population (US 2019)	Weight	Crude Prevalence	Standardized
		Zoster	Population	P_i	$W_i = (P_i) / \Sigma (P_i)$	$Pr_i = (d_i/p_i)*100$	$D_i = Pr_i * W_i$
	Age Groups	d_i	p_i				
Female	20 to 40	3	100	44,001,909	0.178424	3.00	0.5
Female	40 to 60	9	187	41,952,322	0.170113	4.81	0.8
Female	60+	0	28	40,698,389	0.165029	0.00	0.0
Male	20 to 40	0	81	45,308,873	0.183724	0.00	0.0
Male	40 to 60	3	171	40,721,594	0.165123	1.75	0.3
Male	60+	1	24	33,931,020	0.137588	4.17	0.6
Total				246,614,107			
				246,614,107			2.2

Table 6.7. Standardized prevalence of HZ by age and gender in patients with at least one encounter over two years using PROC STDRATE

Age	Sex	Crude Rate	Directly Standardized Rate	Standard Error (stdzd)	CItype	Lower	Upper
20-40	Male	0.00000	0.00000	0.00000	Normal	0.00000	0.00000
40-60	Male	1.75439	0.28969	0.16725	Normal	-0.03812	0.61750
60+	Male	4.16667	0.57328	0.57328	Normal	-0.55033	1.69689
20-40	Female	3.00000	0.53527	0.30904	Normal	-0.07043	1.14098
40-60	Female	4.81283	0.81873	0.27291	Normal	0.28384	1.35362
60+	Female	0.00000	0.00000	0.00000	Normal	0.00000	0.00000

Since estimation of prevalence for each stratum (sex-age) for one single population (zoster sample) using a reference population (e.g., US population) is not part of the output from the STATS option in the STRATA statement of PROC STDRATE and only the crude rates can be calculated, therefore you need to use some extra codes. In fact, the standardized strata rates are each component of the sum in the formula for the overall standardized rates. Their variances are also each component in the sum defining the variance of the overall standardized rates. The code in the fifth section can be used to estimate prevalence and 95% confidence intervals for the strata in Zoster data.

Program 6.6: Descriptive Statistics and Prevalence Estimation for HZ by Sex and Age

```
/*Section 1*/
proc sort data=ehrdata.HZ;
      key patient_id / ascending;
      key HZ / descending;
run;

proc freq data=ehrdata.HZ;
      table sex*age*HZ / norow nocol nocum;
      format age agefmt.;
      where HZ=1;
run;

/*Section 2*/
data HZ;
      input sex $ age $ HZ pyear;
      datalines;
Male 20-40 0 81
Male 40-60 3 171
Male 60+ 1 24
Female 20-40 3 100
Female 40-60 9 187
Female 60+ 0 28
;

/*Section 3*/
data US;
      input sex $ age $ pyear;
      datalines;
Male 20-40 45308873
Male 40-60 40721594
Male 60+ 33931020
```

```
Female 20-40 44001909
Female 40-60 41952322
Female 60+  40698389
;

/*Section 4*/
proc stdrate data=zoster refdata=US method=direct
stat=rate(mult=100);
    population event=zoster total=pyear;
    reference total=pyear;
    strata sex age;
run;

/*Section 5*/
data a;
  merge zoster us(rename=(pyear=refpyear));
  mult=100; alpha=.05; cltype="normal";
  run;
proc sql noprint;
  create table b as
  select age, sex, alpha, cltype,
        mult*zoster/pyear as cruderatej,
        mult*(calculated cruderatej)/pyear as vcrj,
        refpyear/sum(refpyear) as refpropj,
        (calculated refpropj)*(calculated cruderatej) as dsrj,
        (calculated vcrj)*(calculated refpropj)**2 as vdsrj,
        sqrt(calculated vdsrj) as sedsrj,
        (calculated dsrj)+(calculated sedsrj)*quantile('normal',1-(alpha/2)) as upper,
        (calculated dsrj)-(calculated sedsrj)*quantile('normal',1-(alpha/2)) as lower,
        (calculated refpropj)/pyear as wj,
        (calculated wj)**2*(calculated cruderatej)*pyear as vj
    from a;
    quit;
proc print label;
   id age sex;
   var cruderatej dsrj sedsrj cltype lower upper;
   label cruderatej="crude rate" dsrj="directly standardized rate" sedsrj="standard error (stdzd)";
   title "directly standardized strata rates";
   run;
```

In Program 6.6, the STAT= statement specifies the statistic for standardization. STAT=RATE analyzes standardized rates, and STAT=RISK computes standardized risks. Using STAT=RATE(MULT=100) statement, the prevalence will be estimated as percentage by multiplying the rate and the related confidence limits in 100. If you change this statement to STAT=RATE(MULT=10000), the standardized prevalence and its confidence limits will be as the number of cases per 10,000. You can also change the statement to STAT=RISK to get risk ratio instead of prevalence.

As mentioned earlier, since there is only one population here, you can also use Excel or any other spreadsheet software to compute sex-age standardized prevalence within stratified classes. Table 6.6 shows you how you can do that. To calculate standardized prevalence and confidence intervals, you use the same unadjusted prevalence and confidence intervals that you already have in Table 6.2 and substitute them in Table 6.6. Here, only prevalence estimation has been demonstrated. Standardized confidence intervals can be computed by the same method as well. The output from the fifth section and Excel are a little bit different, but the results of prevalence estimation and 95% confidence intervals are the same.

Table 6.7 presents the age-sex standardized prevalence and 95% confidence intervals of zoster. Similar to unadjusted prevalence, the standardized prevalence increases by age in male patients and the prevalence amongst females in 40 to 60 age group is the highest. All standardized prevalence and their confidence intervals are lower than the unadjusted counterparts.

References

Annual Estimates of the Resident Population for Selected Age Groups by Sex for the United States: April 1, 2010 to July 1, 2019 (NC-EST2019-AGESEX). Source: U.S. Census Bureau, Population Division. Release Date: June 2020.

Bains N. 2009. Standardization of Rates. Available at: http://core.apheo.ca/resources/indicators/Standardization%20report_NamBains_FINALMarch16.pdf.

Hudson J. I., Pope H. G. J., Glynn R. J. 2005. *The Cross-Sectional Cohort Study*, Epidemiology: Volume 16 - Issue 3 - p 355–359, https://doi.org/10.1097/01.ede.0000158224.50593.e3.

Kim, Y. S., Seo, H.-M., Bang, C. H., Lee, J. H., Park, Y.-G., Kim, Y. J., Kim, G. M., Park, C. J., Park, H. J., Yu, D. S., Lee, J. Y., & Park, Y. M. 2018. Validation of herpes zoster diagnosis code in the medical record: A retrospective, multicenter study. *Ann Dermatol.* 30(2):253–55. https://doi.org/10.5021/ad.2018.30.2.253.

Queenan J. A., Farahani P., Ehsani M. B., Birtwhistle R. V. 2017. The prevalence and risk for herpes zoster infection in adult patients with diabetes mellitus in the

Canadian Primary Care Sentinel Surveillance Network. *The Canadian Journal of Diabetes.* https://doi.org/10.1016/j.jcjd.2017.10.060.

Schoenbach V. J. 1999. Standardization of rates and ratios. www.epidemiolog.net.

Yuan Y. 2013. Computing Direct and Indirect Standardized Rates and Risks with the STDRATE Procedure. *SAS Global Forum* 2013. Paper 423.

EHRData.Billing and EHRData.HealthCondition tables are based on ICD-10 codes. However, that part of the definition that is related to ICD-9 codes can be converted to ICD-10 codes and the medication information still can be implemented. According to another document that is available from the Ministry of Health in British Colombia (2019), any occurrence of J41 (simple and mucopurulent chronic bronchitis), J42 (unspecified chronic bronchitis), J43 (Emphysema), and J44 (other chronic obstructive pulmonary disease) codes in patient records can be considered as COPD. Although, based on this document, prescribed medication is not part of COPD definition, here you implement the medications that are specified for COPD patients by most physicians as part of disease case definition. Table 7.1 summarizes the case definition that you need to use to classify COPD patients.

Table 7.2. Inclusion and exclusion criteria for COPD case definition

Table	Inclusion	Exclusion
Billing, Health condition, Encounter diagnosis	Patient age must be ≥ 35 years J41 (simple and mucopurulent chronic bronchitis), J42 (unspecified chronic bronchitis), J43 (Emphysema), J44 (other chronic obstructive pulmonary disease)	
OR Medication	R03BB: Anticholinergics, R03AK04: Salbutamol and Sodium Cromoglicate, R03AL: Adrenergics in combination with Anticholinergics including triple combinations with Corticosteroids	Medication alone is not sufficient if patient has Asthma (J45)

7.2.2. Crude Prevalence Estimation

As mentioned earlier in Chapter 6, the best way to start programming for projects that involve prevalence estimation is creating a cohort of patients as denominator first using the fraction of data from the Patient table that represents the contact group. For this study, the fraction of data must include all patients from Jan. 1st, 2019, to Dec. 31st 2020 (two-year contact group). Thus, the denominator of the prevalence equation (equation 1 from Chapter 6) includes all patients who have at least one interaction or visit with their healthcare provider between Jan. 1st 2019 to Dec. 31st 2020. The numerator is the total number of patients who were diagnosed with COPD according to the case definition from Table 7.2.

Thus, the prevalence of COPD as percentage will be:

$$\text{Prevalence of COPD} = \left(\frac{\text{Number of cases with COPD in 2019-2020}}{\text{Total number of patients in 2019-2020}}\right) \times 100 \quad (1)$$

7.3. Analysis and Results

7.3.1. Objective 1: Crude Prevalence Estimation

The following steps provide further details about statistical programming:

1. Sort both the Patient and Encounter tables by their Patient_ID, then merge them, and then create a subset of data for patients that had at least one visit with the primary care provider between Jan. 1st 2019 to Dec. 31st 2020. This subset data is your two-year contact group for the equation (1).
2. Merge the Billing, Encounter_Diagnosis, and Health_Condition tables that contain necessary information for the case definition outlined in the context of Table 7.2. Convert ICD-10 codes for both COPD and asthma to dummy variables. Drop those patients who have been diagnosed with asthma at or after COPD onset and remove duplicate data.
3. Create a subset of data from the Medication table that contains all drug information for COPD patients defined in Table 7.2. Convert ATC codes to dummy variables and remove duplicate data. Merge the product of step 2 with the data set from this step and remove duplicate data.
4. Merge the products of all previous steps and estimate patient age at the onset of COPD using OnsetDate in HealthCondition table. Remove those who were 35 years old or younger at the time of the onset of COPD.
5. Sort data for COPD variable in a descending order, then remove duplicate observations.
6. Estimate total crude prevalence, and prevalence by age and sex.
7. Compute the number of visits for each patient by merging the EHRData.Encounter and the data set that you created from step 5 and compare the average number of visits for patients with and without COPD.

Objective 1: Estimate the crude prevalence of COPD with 95% confidence interval and prevalence by age and sex for those who had at least one visit with their primary health care provider within 2019-2020.

7.3.1.1. Step 1

As mentioned before, you need to merge data from the Patient and Encounter tables first then make a subset of data from patients who had at least one visit with their primary care provider between Jan. 1st 2019 to Dec. 31st 2020. For this step, the match-merge technique, which was explained in Chapter 4, can be utilized to give you cohort records for the next steps. You can use Program 7.1 to carry out the first step.

Program 7.1: Creating a Subset Data Using Match-Merge Technique for Patients who Had at Least One Visit from Jan. 1st, 2019 to Dec. 31st 2020

```
proc sort data=ehrdata.patient;
      by patient_id;
run;

proc sort data=ehrdata.encounter;
      by patient_id;
run;

data patient_encounter (keep=patient_id sex birthday birthmonth birthyear
              encounterdate);
      format EncounterDate mmddyy10.;
      merge ehrdata.patient (in=A) ehrdata.encounter (in=B);
      by patient_id;
      if (A=1 or B=1) then
              output patient_encounter;
run;

data patient_encounter;
      set patient_encounter;
      if '1jan2019'd <=encounterdate<='31dec2020'd;
run;
```

In Program 7.1, data from Patient and Encounter tables are first sorted by Patient_ID, then they are merged, and the subset data is created using two cut off dates.

7.3.1.2. Step 2

Program 7.2 can be used for this part of analysis. Using this program, first you need to merge the Billing, Encounter_Diagnosis, and Health_Condition tables first (Section 1). Recall the difference between different types of match-merging (Table 4.1), since you need all information from patients and you do not want to lose any data, compared to other methods, using "OR" statement for merging data is the best choice here (ABC option from Table 4.1).

Next in the second section, you create two temporary data sets, COPD and Asthma containing their corresponding dummy variables from All_1 table. The COPD data set has records of cases for COPD, and Asthma data set that contains data for asthma cases. You need to convert the ICD-10 codes for these diseases, as specified for these diseases in Table 7.2 to 0 or 1. This part of program is necessary for inclusion and exclusion criteria that are defined in Table 7.2. In this section, you also need to rename DateOfOnset in Asthma data set to something that can be differentiated from the DateOfOnset for COPD (e.g., A_DateOfOnset), otherwise the exclusion criteria cannot be carried out.

In the third section, you will merge the COPD and Asthma data sets and exclude those patients who were diagnosed with asthma at or after COPD onset and you will also remove duplicate data. Although exclusion criterion should be implemented on medication table, but if it is executed at this step will make the programming more efficient with less coding.

Program 7.2: Creation of COPD Data Set
and Exclusion of Asthma Patients

```
/*Section 1*/
proc sort data=ehrdata.billing;
      by patient_id;
run;

proc sort data=ehrdata.encounterdiagnosis;
      by patient_id;
run;

proc sort data=ehrdata.healthcondition;
      by patient_id;
run;

data all_1 (drop=diagnosiscodetype_calc diagnosistext_calc);
```

```
        format dateofonset mmddyy10.;
        merge ehrdata.billing (in=A)
ehrdata.encounterdiagnosis (in=B)
              ehrdata.healthcondition (in=C);
        by patient_id;
        if (A=1 or B=1 or C=1) then
              output all_1;
run;

/*Section 2*/
data COPD;
      set all_1;

      if (substr(diagnosiscode_calc, 1, 3)) in ("J41",
"J42", "J43", "J44") then
            COPD=1;
      else
            COPD=0;
run;

data COPD (keep=patient_id COPD dateofonset);
      set COPD;

proc sort data=COPD;
      key patient_id /ascending;
      key COPD/descending;
run;

Data COPD;
      Set COPD;
      by patient_id;

      if first. patient_id;
run;

data asthma;
      set all_1;

      if (substr(diagnosiscode_calc, 1, 3)) in ("J45") then
            asthma=1;
      else
            asthma=0;
      rename dateofonset=a_dateofonset;
run;
data asthma (keep=patient_id asthma a_dateofonset);
      set asthma;

proc sort data=asthma;
      key patient_id /ascending;
```

```
              key asthma/descending;
run;

Data asthma;
        Set asthma;
        by patient_id;

        if first. patient_id;
run;

/*Section 3*/
data all_2;
        merge COPD (in=A) Asthma (in=B);
        by patient_id;

        if (A=1 or B=1) then
                output all_2;
run;

data all_2;
        set all_2;

        if COPD=1 and Asthma=0 then
                COPD1=1;
        else if COPD=1 and Asthma=1 and
a_dateofonset>dateofonset then
                COPD1=1;
        else
                COPD1=0;
run;

data all_2 (keep=dateofonset patient_id COPD1);
        set all_2;

data all_2;
        set all_2;
        rename COPD1=COPD;
run;
```

7.3.1.3. Step 3

In the first section of Program 7.3, you will create a temporary data set from the EHRData.Medication table (Medication) then you merge it with the data set from Step 2. In the next section of this program, you create a new dummy variable (COPD1) by converting all ATC drug codes that are prescribed to COPD patients and specified in Table 7.2 to 0 or 1. The StartDate >= DateOfOnset statement limits the COPD medications at or after onset of the

Prevalence Estimation for Chronic Diseases   111

disease and not before. At the end of this step, you integrate both COPD and COPD1 variables into one single variable (Disease) that represents the presence or absence of COPD disease, and you will also drop the unnecessary variables. Removal of duplicate observations for the Disease variable should be done in the next step after merging the product of this step with that of Step 1 (two-year contact group).

Program 7.3: Creation of Medication Data Set for COPD Patients

```
/*Section 1*/
data medication (keep=patient_id startdate code_calc
datecreated);
        set ehrdata.medication;
run;

proc sort data=medication;
        by patient_id;
run;

data all_3;
        merge all_2 (in=A) medication (in=B);
        by patient_id;

        if (A=1 or B=1) then
                output all_3;
run;

/*Section 2*/
data all_3;
        format DateOfOnset mmddyy10.;
        format DateCreated mmddyy10.;
        set all_3;

        if (index(code_calc, "R03BB") or index(code_calc,
"R03SAK04") or
                index(code_calc, " R03AL")) and startdate
>=dateofonset then
                        COPD1=1;
        else
                        COPD1=0;
run;
data all_3;
        set all_3;
        if COPD=1 or COPD1=1 then
                disease=1;
        else
```

```
                disease=0;
run;

data all_3 (keep=patient_id dateofonset disease);
      set all_3;
run;
```

7.3.1.4. Step 4

In the first section of this step, you will compute patient age at the onset of COPD diagnosis using the OnsetDate variable (Program 7.4). Next, you will remove all unnecessary variables, then you will restrict your analysis to those patients with 35 years old or older and you will also rename the disease variable to COPD. In the second section of the same step, by sorting COPD variable in a descending order and by removing duplicate observations, the data set will be ready for prevalence estimation.

Program 7.4: Estimation of Patient Age at Onset of COPD Disease

```
/*Section 1*/
data all_4 (keep=patient_ID sex BirthDay BirthMonth BirthYear disease
            dateofonset encounterdate);
      merge patient_encounter (in=A) all_3 (in=B);
      by patient_id;

      if (A=1) then
            output all_4;
run;

data all_4;
      format dateofonset mmddyy10.;
      format encounterdate mmddyy10.;
      set all_4;
      birthdate=mdy(birthmonth, birthday, birthyear);
      format birthdate mmddyy10.;
      idate=(dateofonset);
      bdate=(birthdate);
      ageint=idate-bdate;
      age=ageint/365.2422;


      format age 6.1;
run;
```

Prevalence Estimation for Chronic Diseases

```
data all_4 (drop=encounterdate birthday birthmonth birthyear
dateofonset
            birthdate idate bdate ageint);
      set all_4;
      where age>=35;
      rename disease=COPD;
run;

/*Section 2*/
proc sort data=all_4;
      key patient_id / ascending;
      key COPD / descending;
run;

data ehrdata.all_4;
      set all_4;
      by patient_id;

      if first.patient_id;
run;
```

7.3.1.5. Step 5

Using Program 7.5 you can estimate the descriptive statistics of age by gender for patients with or without COPD, total crude prevalence, and the prevalence of the disease by age and gender for patients with at least one encounter over two years.

Program 7.5: Descriptive Statistics for Age and Prevalence Estimation for COPD Patients

```
proc format;
      value agefmt 35-<50='A: < 50'
50-<65='B: 50 to 65'
65-high='C: 65+';
run;

proc means data= ehrdata.all_4 maxdec=1 mean clm range std;
      class sex;
      var age;
      where COPD=1;
      title "age characteristics of patients with COPD";
run;
```

```
proc means data= ehrdata.all_4 maxdec=1 mean clm range std;
      class sex;
      var age;
      where COPD=0;
      title "age characteristics of patients without COPD";
run;

proc means data= ehrdata.all_4 maxdec=3 mean clm;
      var COPD;
run;

proc means data= ehrdata.all_4 maxdec=3 mean clm;
      class age sex;
      var COPD;
      format age agefmt.;
run;
```

In Program 7.5, first you introduce the age category that you need by using PROC FORMAT. Then you estimate several statistics including mean and confidence limits for patient age for those with or without COPD. Then, you will estimate the total prevalence of COPD and its 95% confidence interval and the prevalence by gender and age. By multiplying the prevalence and its confidence limits in 100, you will get prevalence as percentage.

Table 7.3 shows age characteristics for patients with or without COPD. According to this table, the average age for female patients with COPD is 50.6, which is higher than average age for male patients which is 48.0 years old. The age difference between males and females is very small for those without COPD.

Table 7.3. Age characteristics of patients with or without COPD

Sex	N	Mean	Lower 95% CL for Mean	Upper 95% CL for Mean	Range	Std Dev
With COPD						
Female	17	50.6	47.4	53.7	25.8	6.1
Male	23	48.0	44.8	51.2	28.7	7.4
Without COPD						
Female	244	48.7	47.6	49.7	34.7	8.2
Male	218	48.3	47.2	49.4	34.3	8.4

Table 7.4. Crude prevalence of COPD by age and gender in patients with at least one encounter over two years

Age	Sex	N Obs	Prevalence (%)	Lower 95% CL for Mean	Upper 95% CL for Mean
A: < 50	Female	156	5.1	1.6	8.6
	Male	139	9.4	4.5	14.3
B: 50 to 65	Female	100	9.0	3.3	14.7
	Male	94	9.6	3.5	15.6
C: 65+	Female	5	0	.	.
	Male	8	12.5	-17.1	42.1

According to the third section of Program 6.5, the overall crude prevalence of COPD for those 35 years old or older and with at least one encounter during 2019–2020 is 8.0% (95% CI: 5.6, 10.3). Table 7.4 demonstrate the age and sex stratified prevalence of COPD in the database. The prevalence increases by age in male patients. The prevalence of COPD is the highest amongst male patients in the 60+ age group. Again, here the lower bounds of confidence intervals with negative signs can be replaced with zero as the rates cannot be negative. The group categories that their confidence interval includes the null value (0) are considered as non-significant.

Objective 2: Estimate the average number of total healthcare visits that COPD patients had during 2019-2020 and compare the result with those who do not have the disease.

7.3.2. Objective 2: Number of Healthcare Visits

In this part, you investigate the effect of COPD as a chronic disease on healthcare visits and you identify characteristics of patients associated with frequent visits. Using Program 7.6, you can estimate the total number of visits for each patient. In the first section, you make a temporary data set (Visits) from EHRData.Encounter. Then, you remove all possible duplicate encounter dates for each patient. Next, you calculate the total number of visits for each person, followed by dropping unnecessary variables, sorting Visit variable in a descending order, and removing duplicate data. In the second section, you merge the product of the first section with all_4 data set, which contains COPD observations. In the third section, you will estimate the average of healthcare visits for patient with or without COPD and its 95% confidence interval by sex and age stratification (Table 7.5).

Program 7.6: Number of Visit Estimation for COPD Patients

```
/*Section 1*/
data visits;
        set ehrdata.encounter (drop=network datecreated);
Run;

proc sort data=visits nodupkey;
        key patient_id encounterdate;
run;

data visits;
        set visits;
        by patient_id;

        if first.patient_id then
                visit=1;
        else
                visit+1;
run;

data visits (drop=encounterdate);
        set visits;
Run;

proc sort data=visits;
        key patient_id / ascending;
        key visit / descending;
run;

data visits;
        Set visits;
        by patient_id;

        if first. patient_id;
run;

/*Section 2*/
data all_visits;
        merge ehrdata.all_4 (in=A) visits (in=B);
        by patient_id;

        if (A=1) then
                output all_visits;
```

```
run;

/*Section 3*/
proc means data=all_visits mean maxdec=1 clm;
    var visit;
    where COPD=1;
    title "average number of visits of patients with COPD";
run;

proc means data=all_visits mean maxdec=1 clm;
    var visit;
    where COPD=0;
    title "average number of visits of patients without COPD";
run;

proc means data=all_visits mean maxdec=1 clm;
    class age sex;
    var visit;
    where COPD=1;
    format age agefmt.;
    title "average number of visits of patients with COPD by age and sex";
run;

proc means data=all_visits mean maxdec=1 clm;
    class age sex;
    var visit;
    where COPD=0;
    format age agefmt.;
    title "average number of visits of patients without COPD by age and sex";
run;
```

Table 7.5. Average number of visits for patients with COPD by age and sex in patients with at least one encounter over two years

Age	Sex	N Obs	Mean	Lower 95% CL for Mean	Upper 95% CL for Mean
A: < 50	Female	8	233.4	231.1	235.7
	Male	13	234.8	233.5	236.2
B: 50 to 65	Female	9	235.1	233.5	236.7
	Male	9	236.0	234.5	237.5
C: 65+	Male	1	234.0	.	.

Table 7.6. Average number of visits for patients without COPD by age and sex in patients with at least one encounter over two years

Age	Sex	N Obs	Mean	Lower 95% CL for Mean	Upper 95% CL for Mean
A: < 50	Female	148	235.2	234.8	235.6
	Male	126	235.3	234.9	235.7
B: 50 to 65	Female	91	235.3	234.8	235.8
	Male	85	235.4	234.9	236.0
C: 65+	Female	5	235.6	233.7	237.5
	Male	7	235.1	232.8	237.5

According to the results of this part of the analysis, the average number of visits by COPD patients during 2019–2020 is 234.9 (95% CI: 234.1-235.6), and for patients without COPD, it is 235.3 (95% CI: 235.1-235.5). Therefore, there is no significant difference between patients with or without COPD for healthcare visits. According to Tables 7.5 and 7.6, there is also no difference by age and sex of patients for healthcare visits.

References

BC Chronic Disease and Selected Procedure Case Definitions. 2019. Chronic Disease Information Working Group, British Colombia Ministry of Health. Available at: http://www.bccdc.ca/resource-gallery/Documents/Chronic-Disease-Dashboard/chronic-obstructive-pulmonary-disease.pdf.

Green, M. E., Natajaran, N., O'Donnell, D. E., Williamson, T., Kotecha, J., Khan, S., & Cave, A. 2015. Chronic obstructive pulmonary disease in primary care: an epidemiologic cohort study from the Canadian Primary Care Sentinel Surveillance Network. *CMAJ Open.* vol. 3 no. 1 E15-E22. https://doi.org/10.9778/cmajo.20140040.

Chapter 8

Disease Case Validation

Abstract

Data derived from EHR databases are becoming increasingly popular in medical research, surveillance, and decision support systems. To computerize medical information, healthcare practitioners need to type explanatory text for the diagnosis or symptoms and select the most applicable entry from a drop-down list of possible choices. Other information that is entered into EHR system are prescriptions with dosages, records of weight and height, blood pressure, vaccinations, laboratory test results, and referral. The validity of research utilizing this information depends on the quality and quantity of data recorded. It is not unusual that, for example, diseases may become misdiagnosed or miscoded or medications are coded wrong. Consequently, patient classification and all statistical parameters related to the classification such as prevalence of a disease that are estimated using information from EHR data may possibly become different from the true statistical parameters of the population due to false positive or false negative records. Not to mention that misclassified data and systematic errors in EHR can lead to inferential errors too. To examine this possibility and broaden the usability of EHR data, researchers need to assess and measure the validity of certain electronic diagnoses such as patient classification for diseases, particularly for disease case definition by conducting validation studies.

8.1. Objectives

The purpose of this chapter is to provide a summary of programming methods that are used to validate case definitions in primary care EHR data using gold standard validation. For hands-on experience, the final results of the classification for COPD patients from Chapter 7 will be cross validated with a gold standard data set.

8.2. Methodology

There are several methods to test the validity of EHR diagnostic algorithms. Sometimes these methods are divided into external and internal validation (Herrett et al., 2010). External validation requires reliable (standard) external reference, which is called the "gold standard" for comparison. This method is resource-intensive, and the comparison can be quantified using some precision metrics such as sensitivity and specificity. Internal validation does not need any standard reference, which will therefore not be able to quantify the test measures. There are also other methods to categorize validation techniques such as questionnaires for healthcare practitioners or patients, manual validation of physical records, validation of machine-learning algorithms and so on (Nissen et al., 2019). The selection of validation technique depends on the nature of a study including the objectives of the research project and available resources including access to data. The statistical analysis and information about programming in this chapter can be used to implement any type of validation technique. For simplicity, gold standard validation is considered as the default option for validation in the remainder of this chapter.

8.2.1. Precision Metrics

The results of the EHR diagnosis algorithm for patient classification using a rule-based system can be cross validated by a gold standard data set. The precision metrics resulting from cross-validations are expressed by accuracy and other relevant statistics that are calculated from a confusion matrix (contingency table) for binary classifier (Table 8.1).

Table 8.1. The 2 × 2 contingency table displays the performance evaluation by comparison between classified values from a gold standard system and observed values from the rule-based system

Classified by Gold Standard	Classified by Rule-based System		Row Total
	No	Yes	
No	TN	FP (α=Type I error)	
Yes	FN (β=Type II error)	TP	
Column Total			

Disease Case Validation

$$\text{Accuracy} = \frac{TP+TN}{TP+TN+FP+FN} \quad (1)$$

$$\text{Sensitivity} = \frac{TP}{TP+FN} \quad (2)$$

$$\text{Specificity} = \frac{TN}{TN+FP} \quad (3)$$

$$PPV = \frac{TP}{TP+FP} \quad (4)$$

$$NPV = \frac{TN}{TN+FN} \quad (5)$$

$$\text{Kappa (Cohen's)} = \frac{P_o - P_e}{1 - P_e} \quad (6)$$

where TP, TN, FP, FN, PPV and NPV are true positives, true negatives, false positives, false negatives, positive predictive value (precision), and negative predictive value, respectively. TP involves cases in which you classify patients as Yes for a disease using rule-based system, and in fact they have the disease. TN is cases where you classified patients as No for a disease, and they do not have the disease. FP are cases that you classified patients as Yes for a disease, but they do not actually have the disease. This is also called a Type I error (α). FN is the cases that are classified as No, but they have the disease. This is also called a Type II error (β).

Accuracy is the most intuitive metric, and it is the ratio of correctly classified cases to the total cases. When the numbers of FP and FN are almost the same and accuracy level is relatively high, the accuracy alone will be a good measurement to confirm that the classification algorithm is working properly. But when the numbers of FP and FN are not the same, then having a high accuracy alone is not enough and other metrics should be taken into consideration.

The most common metric is sensitivity (recall). It is especially important when you really need to correctly predict the cases in the true class.

PPV or precision is the ratio of the positive cases that are predicted correctly relative to all the positive predictions. This metric is particularly important when the number of positive cases are very low, for example in rare disease cases.

Specificity is a metric that gives you the true negative rate, and it is especially important when the true prediction of negative cases is more important than positive cases.

The NPV is the ratio of the negative cases that are predicted correctly relative to all the negative predictions.

Finally, Cohen's Kappa is a measure of how well the classifier algorithm performed classification compared to chance. In Kappa formula, P_o is the relative observed agreement among raters (equal with accuracy), and P_e is the hypothetical probability of chance agreement.

8.3. Analysis and Results

8.3.1. Objective: Cross-validation for COPD Classified Cases

Suppose after creating the EHRData.All_4 data set, which contains all patients with and without COPD cases using the COPD case definition and the algorithm that you created for patient classification, you want to assess whether the case definition for COPD is classifying positive and negative cases properly or not. Suppose also you hired an independent chart reviewer to audit all available patients (n=502) in the EHRData.All_4 data set using the SOAP (the Subjective, Objective, Assessment and Plan) notes, handwritings, lab test results, and other available and valid information. Then after a while, the reviewer returns with a data set that contains all patients (assuming that there were no missing data) with true information about their COPD diagnosis. Let's assume that the EHRData.Copd_gold_standard data set is the data set that your chart auditor created, and you want to cross-validate the classified cases in EHRData.All_4 with the gold standard. Program 8.1 can be used to quantify the validity of the COPD classification that was carried out in Chapter 7.

Program 8.1: Cross-validation of COPD Data with Gold Standard

```
/*Section 1*/
data both (drop=age sex);
      merge ehrdata.copd_gold_standard(in=A)
ehrdata.all_4(in=B);
      by patient_id;
```

Disease Case Validation

```
                if a=1 then
                        output both;
        Run;

        proc freq data=both order=data;
                tables COPDg*COPD/ norow nocol nocum;
        run;

        data validation;
                input gold_std$ role_based$ count;
                datalines;
        0  0   446
        0  1   9
        1  0   16
        1  1   31
        ;

        /*Section 2*/

                title 'Sensitivity';

        proc freq data=validation;
                where gold_std="1";
                weight count;
                tables role_based / binomial(level="1");
                exact binomial;
        run;

        title 'Specificity';

        proc freq data=validation;
                where gold_std="0";
                weight count;
                tables role_based / binomial(level="0");
                exact binomial;
        run;

        title 'Positive predictive value';

        proc freq data=validation;
                where role_based="1";
                weight count;
                tables gold_std / binomial(level="1");
                exact binomial;
        run;

        title 'Negative predictive value';

        proc freq data=validation;
```

```
            where role_based="0";
            weight count;
            tables gold_std / binomial(level="1");
            exact binomial;
run;

title 'Accuracy';

data acc;
       set validation;

       if (role_based and gold_std) or
             (not role_based and not gold_std) then
                  acc="1";
       else
                  acc="0";
run;

proc freq;
       weight count;
       tables acc / binomial(level="1");
       exact binomial;
run;

ods graphics on;
title 'Kappa';

proc freq data=validation order=data;
       tables role_based*gold_std / norow nocol nopercent
agree;
       test kappa;
       weight count;
run;

ods graphics off;
```

In the first section of Program 8.1, you merge the EHRData.Copd_gold_standard data with the EHRData.All_4 table. Then using PROC FREQ, you create a temporary small data set (Validation). The Validation data set has all the elements of Table 8.1 and can be utilized for the second section of the program and for estimation of all precision metrics from cross-validation. Table 8.2 reports the results of performance evaluation of the COPD classification by comparison between classified cases from the EHR rule-based algorithm and observed values from chart audit. According to the table, there were 477 (95.0%) correct classifications (446 cases for "No" and

31 cases for "Yes", along the diagonal) and 25 (5.0%) incorrect classifications (9 cases for "No" and 16 cases for "Yes", along the vertical).

Table 8.2. The 2 × 2 contingency table displays the performance evaluation for COPD classification by comparison between classified values by chart audit (gold standard) and observed values from the rule-based system

Classified by Gold Standard	Classified Observations by Rule-based System		
	No	Yes	Row Total
No	446	9	455
Yes	16	31	47
Column Total	462	40	502

According to the results of Program 8.1 (Table 8.3), the overall sensitivity, specificity, positive predictive value, negative predictive value, accuracy, and Kappa of the COPD classification are 0.66 (0.52, 0.80), 0.98 (0.97, 0.99), 0.78 (0.65, 0.90), 0.97 (0.95, 0.98), 0.95 (0.93, 0.97) and 0.69 (0.57, 0.80), respectively.

Table 8.3. Precision metrics for COPD classification by comparison between classified values by chart audit (gold standard) and observed values from the rule-based system

Precision Metrics	Test Measurements with 95% CI
Sensitivity	0.66 (0.52, 0.80)
Specificity	0.98 (0.97, 0.99)
PPV	0.78 (0.65, 0.90)
NPV	0.97 (0.95, 0.98)
Accuracy	0.95 (0.93, 0.97)
Cohen's Kappa	0.69 (0.57, 0.80)

In addition to the metrics of Table 8.3, you can also estimate other accuracy parameters such as the false positive probability for both columns and rows in Table 8.2 and false negative probability, the proportion of true positive results that have a negative test result for the column and row of the same table using Program 8.1.

Program 8.2: False Positive and False Negative Probabilities Resulting from Cross-validation of COPD Data with Gold Standard

```
proc freq data=validation;
    where role_based="0";
    weight count;
    tables gold_std / binomial(level="0");
    exact binomial;
run;

title 'False Positive Probability (Col)';

proc freq data=validation;
    where gold_std="0";
    weight count;
    tables role_based / binomial(level="1");
    exact binomial;
run;

title 'False Positive Probability (Row)';

proc freq data=validation;
    where role_based="1";
    weight count;
    tables gold_std / binomial(level="0");
    exact binomial;
run;

title 'False Negative Probability (Col)';

proc freq data=validation;
    where gold_std="1";
    weight count;
    tables role_based / binomial(level="0");
    exact binomial;
run;

title 'False Negative Probability (Row)';
```

8.3.2. Sample Size Calculation

In Section 8.3.1, all available patients (n=502) from EHRData.All_4 data set were audited for performance assessment. In actual practice, using all available data can be realistic only when the sample size is small or when there are no limitations on resources, budget, human resource, ethical approval and so on. But most of the time due to some limitations, you can only use a small fraction of the data for cross-validation. In such cases, to accommodate your research objectives and to avoid any problem, sample size needs to be calculated precisely and wisely with respect to Type I error, Type II error, the rate of positive cases and the statistical power. SAS has two procedures for sample size calculation. PROC POWER and PROC GLMPOWER perform prospective power and sample size estimations. "Prospective" indicates that the analysis refers to planning for a future study and not to a retrospective analysis. The power and sample size calculations for a past study are not supported by these procedures. The POWER procedure covers a variety of statistical analyses such as t-tests, equivalence tests, and confidence intervals for means, multiple regression and so on. The GLMPOWER procedure focuses on power analysis for more complex linear models, for example when between/within-subject contrasts for multivariate models are important or when "what-if" is part of analysis to assess sensitivity of the power or sample size. For a comprehensive information about these procedures refers to Power and Sample Size in SAS/STAT Software.[1]

Unfortunately, to the best knowledge of the author, currently SAS does not have any specific method for sample size or power calculations for cross-validation study. However, PROC POWER for a t-test or ANOVA can be tailored for sample size calculation of cross-validation projects. Program 8.3 gives you sample size for two groups of COPD patients (male and female) using the ANOVA method. First, you estimate the COPD mean values and standard deviations by sex. Then by substituting these numbers in PROC POWER, you calculate the sample size. In the PROC POWER statement, the minimum and maximum power (1-β) are considered 0.5 and 0.99, respectively, and the Type I error or alpha is equal to 0.05. The NFRACTIONAL statement allows fractional sample size estimation (first section).

Program 8.3: Sample Size for Two Groups of COPD Patients Using the ANOVA Method

```
/* Section 1*/
proc means data=ehrdata.all_4 mean std maxdec=3;
      class sex;
      var COPD;
```

---

[1] https://support.sas.com/rnd/app/stat/procedures/PowerSampleSize.html#power.

```
title "COPD Mean and Standard Deviation by Sex";
run;

ods noproctitle;
ods graphics / imagemap=on;

proc power;
    onewayanova test=overall groupmeans=(0.065 0.095)
stddev=0.247 0.294 power=0.5 0.99 alpha=0.05 nfractional
npergroup=.;
    plot x=power min=0.5 max=0.99;
run;
ods graphics off;

/* Section 2*/
proc power;
    twosamplemeans test=diff sides=2 groupmeans=(0.065
0.095) stddev=0.247 0.294
         power=0.8 alpha=0.05 nfractional npergroup=.;
    plot x=power;
run;
```

By defining the minimum and maximum values for power, you can obtain the graph that displays power curve, which you can then use it as a guidance for the selection of the best sample size. According to Figure 8.1, a sample size of equal or bigger than 1066 and 1509 is needed to achieve a power of at least 0.8 for female and male groups, respectively. Using the two-sample t-test code from the second section of Program 8.3 will give you the same results.

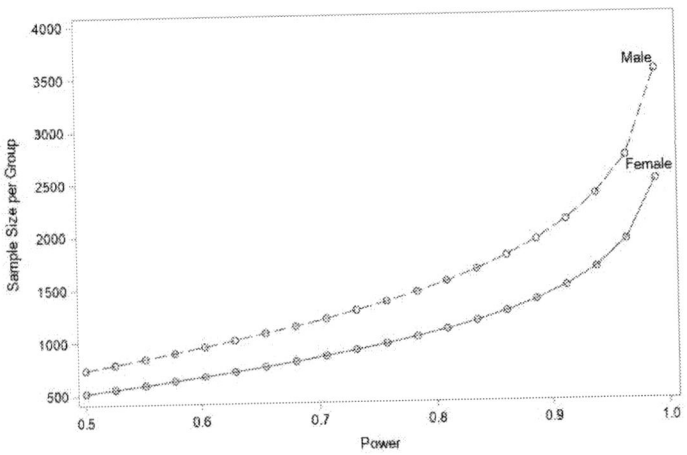

Figure 8.1. Sample size for COPD cross-validation by group (sex).

References

Herrett, E., Thomas, S. L., Schoonen, W. M., Smeeth, L., & Hall, A. J. 2010. Validation and validity of diagnoses in the General Practice Research Database: a systematic review. *Br J Clin Pharmacol.* 69: 4–14.

Nissen, F., Quint, J. K., Morales, D. R., & Douglas, I. J., 2019. How to validate a diagnosis recorded in electronic health records. *Breathe.* 15: 64–68.

Chapter 9

Multiple Logistic Regression

Abstract

In clinical practice, prediction models can reduce the burden of a disease by assisting patients and their health service providers with a diagnostic or a prognostic outcome or with the classification of patients according to their risk assessment (Steyerberg, 2009). Choosing a correct model depends on the outcome variable, the combination of input variables, and whether the input variables are fixed effects or random effects. When the response outcome is not continuous like in many clinical studies, error terms in models are not normally distributed and a normal distribution function is not appropriate for making the model. In such cases, the logistic distribution function which is like the normal distribution function can be applied.

This chapter discusses the process of developing Multiple Logistic Regression (MLR) models for healthcare data as well as the presentation of corresponding results. The purpose of an MLR model is to obtain the best fitting and simplest equation that predicts the probability of a value of Y (the outcome or dependent variable) as a function of the $X_1, ..., X_n$ (covariates, predictors, explanatory or independent variables). After creating such an equation, you can then plug the values of independent variables into the equation for a new individual and estimate the probability of occurrence of a specific value of the dependent variable. The difference between an MLR model and the linear regression model is that in MLR the outcome variable is binary (or dichotomous). MLR and, in general, logistic regression are also simple supervised machine learning algorithms that are used to predict or classify the probability of a binary outcome 1 (yes/true) or 0 (no/false). An MLR model uses the sigmoid (also known as logistic) function and can employ different types of predictors such as continuous, discrete, and categorical variables.

In SAS, PROC LOGISTIC is the standard and is specifically designed for fitting logistic regression models, but other procedures such as PHREG, GENMOD, GLIMMIX, NLINMIX, NLMIXED and HPGENSELECT can also be used. Application of any of these methods depends on the data and on the interpretation of parameters.

Among these procedures, PROC LOGISTIC and PROC GENMOD are more popular than others. PROC GENMOD has some advantages over PROC LOGISTIC for creating MLR. In PROC GENMOD, unlike its counterpart, you can use a class statement for specifying categorical variables, which will omit the necessity of constructing indicator variables in advance. Interactions between two or more variables can easily be included by specifying statements such as variable1|variable2. Unlike PROC LOGISTIC that requires explanatory variables to be an integer, in PROC GENMOD the response variable or the explanatory variable can be character too. Moreover, PROC GENMOD can handle the analysis of correlated data with underlying distribution from exponential family. PROC GLIMMIX, which is relatively a new SAS procedure and has almost all properties of GENMOD procedure, can also be used to fit a Generalized Linear Mixed model.

In addition to these procedures, PROC HPGENSELECT can also be applied for categorical data. PROC HPGENSELECT is a high-performance technique that provides model fitting for generalized linear models. You can use this procedure to fit models for data with standard distributions from the exponential family, such as the Gaussian, binomial, negative binomial, Poisson, and Tweedie distributions. PROC HPGENSELECT also fits multinomial models for ordinal and nominal outcomes, and it can also fit zero-inflated Poisson (ZIP) model for count data and the estimation of the parameters is carried out using maximum likelihood techniques.

Moreover, it can also perform variable selection using forward, backward, stepwise, and LASSO (Least Absolute Shrinkage and Selection Operator) techniques. PROC HPGENSELECT is especially helpful for large-data tasks, such as predictive model building, model fitting, and scoring.[1]

9.1. Objectives

The objective of this chapter is to find the simplest and the best fitting model describing the relationship between an outcome as a dependent variable and predictors using PROC HPGENSELECT.

---

[1] For more information about PROC HPGENSELECT, see the SAS/STAT® 14.1 User's Guide.

9.2. Methodology

9.2.1. Data Set

Data from Sashelp.Birthwgt will be used to extract information about infant mortality in 2003 in the USA. The data set contains 100,000 random observations from the US National Center for Health Statistics. Each observation includes infant death within one year of birth, birth weight, maternal smoking and drinking behavior, and other characteristics of the mother. If we assume that each observation is carried out independently and if for the combination of all independent variables there is a constant probability for infant death, then the random variable Death follows a Bernoulli distribution where the success probability is a function of all predictors in Table 9.1. Hence, Death is considered as a binary response variable and the rest are categorical variables with the fix effects. You need to select the best independent variables and all two-way interactions by the LASSO selection technique using PROC HPGENSELECT.

Table 9.1. Alphabetic list of variables and attributes for infant mortality data in 2003

Variable	Type	Length
AgeGroup	Num	8
Death	Char	3
Drinking	Char	3
LowBirthWgt	Char	3
Married	Char	3
Race	Char	9
Smoking	Char	3
SomeCollege	Char	3

9.3. Analysis and Results

9.3.1. MLR Model Fit Using PROC HPGENSELECT

In the first section of Program 9.1, you make a temporary data set from sashelp.birthwgt, then you add ID variable for observations in the data set. Having ID for observations is necessary if you need to make predictions based on the constructed model. Then in the second section, the dependency of the probability of death for infants is modeled as a function of birth weight, maternal smoking and drinking behavior, and other attributes of the mother, plus their two-way interactions.

Program 9.1: Variable Selection and Model Fitting for Infant Mortality Data Using PROC HPGENSELECT

```
/*Section 1*/
data birthwgt;
    set sashelp.birthwgt;
    id=_n_;
run;

/*Section 2*/
proc hpgenselect data=sashelp.birthwgt ;
    partition fraction(validate=0.15 test=0.15 seed=255)
;
    class married agegroup race lowbirthwgt smoking drinking somecollege /
        param=glm;
    model death(event="Yes")=married | agegroup | race | lowbirthwgt | smoking | drinking | somecollege @2
    / dist=binary link=logit;
run;
```

In this program, the PARTITION statement specifies how observations in the input data set should be divided into subsets for model training, validation, and testing. When there is enough data, by partitioning data into three parts (training, validation, and test data) for a model fit or during the model selection process, models can be fitted, and attributes can be selected based on the training data. After fitting the model, the validation data set can be used to assess how the selected model can be generalized on holdout test data that played no role in selecting the model. In Program 9.1, the data set randomly divided about 15% for validation and 15% for testing and the rest (about 70%) for training. Currently, the HPGENSELECT procedure does not use validation data, hence the validation and test data subsets are the same.

The SEED= option in the program defines a random integer to start the partitioning of data randomly for training, testing, and validation. By using the same number in future, you get the same results for analysis. In the lack of seed number, the seed is generated by the time of day from computer's clock.

The PARAM=GLM statement that indicates the method that is requested for parameterization of CLASS variables, can be dropped from the program, because like PROC GENMOD, the default parameterization in the HPGENSELECT procedure is GLM parameterization. You can also change the parameterization method by specifying the PARAM= option. EVENT="Yes" specifies the event category and modeling of the probability of "Yes" for the binary outcome of Death. When there are more than two response categories, the EVENT= option has no effect.

The model information table indicates that the data are modeled as binary distributed with a logit link function (Table 9.2). The logit link is the default function for binary and binomial data. PROC HPGENSELECT used a ridged Newton-Raphson algorithm to estimate the parameters of the binary model.

Table 9.2. Model information for infant mortality in 2003

Data Source	SASHELP.BIRTHWGT
Response Variable	Death
Class Parameterization	GLM
Distribution	Binary
Link Function	Logit
Optimization Technique	Newton-Raphson with Ridging
Seed	255

The next tables, Tables 9.3 and 9.4, show how observations including the response variable in the input Birthwgt data set were partitioned into separate subsets for model training, validation, and testing.

Table 9.3. Number of observations for infant mortality based on data partitioning

Description	Total	Training	Validation	Testing
Number of Observations Read	100000	69984	15081	14935
Number of Observations Used	93292	65306	14067	13919

Table 9.4. Response profile for infant mortality based on data partitioning

Ordered Value	Death	Total Frequency	Training	Validation	Testing
1	No	92765	64943	13974	13848
2	Yes	527	363	93	71

Table 9.5 presents the fit statistics for infant mortality for the saturated (full) model. The value of the -2 times of log-likelihood function equals 3537.65, 956.52, and 749.45 for the Training, Validation, and Test data sets, respectively. Additional fit statistics AIC (Akaike's information criterion), AICC (small-sample bias-corrected version of AIC), and BIC (Bayesian criterion) are also given, in which "smaller is better" applies for all of them except for the Log Likelihood, which in this case the bigger is better. The goal is finding the coefficients (βs) that maximize the Log Likelihood.

Table 9.5. Fit statistics for infant mortality full model in 2003

Fit Statistics	Training	Validation	Testing
-2 Log Likelihood	3537.65	956.52	749.45
AIC (smaller is better)	3657.65	1076.52	869.45
AICC (smaller is better)	3657.76	1077.04	869.98
BIC (smaller is better)	4202.86	1529.61	1321.91
Pearson Chi-Square	66082	26616	16536
Pearson Chi-Square/DF	1.0128	1.9002	1.1931
Average Square Error	0.005329	0.006422	0.004965

The **Parameter Estimates** table in the output shows the estimates and standard errors of the model effects. Since this table was too large, it was not presented here; however, the summary will be reported briefly. According to this table, the main effects of Race and LowBirthWgt are significant, and the rest are non-significant. The interaction between AgeGroup*Race, Married*LowBirthWgt, and Married*SomeCollege are also significant at least at $\alpha=0.05$ level.

In model building when there is a large data with many predictors, the most difficult task is eliminating unnecessary variables and keeping only those that fit with the model best. Furthermore, using all variables can increase the risk of over fitting the model. That is why fitting any model starts with a selection process. The model that was created in Program 9.1 is called the full or saturated model. The syntax from Program 9.2 can be used to select independent variables and fit the model with the best predictors.

Program 9.2: Variable Selection and Model Fitting for Infant Mortality Data Using LASSO Technique

```
proc hpgenselect data=birthwgt ;
      partition fraction(validate=0.30  seed=255) ;
```

```
        class married agegroup race lowbirthwgt smoking
drinking somecollege /
            param=glm;
        model death(event="Yes")=married | agegroup | race |
lowbirthwgt | smoking | drinking | somecollege @2
            / dist=binary link=logit;
        selection method=lasso(stop=sbc choose=sbc)
details=all ;
        id id;
        output out=out xbeta predicted=pred;
        run;
```

The SELECTION statement performs model selection by evaluating the effects that should be added to or dropped from the model according to guidelines which are defined by SELECTION METHOD functions (CHOOSE=SBC) and model selection methods. In Program 9.2, the selection of attributes that are most relevant in relation to infant mortality forecasting in the Birthwgt dataset is also investigated by LASSO selection technique (Tibshirani, 1996) and lowest Schwarz Bayesian Information Criterion (SBC) (Schwarz, 1978). PROC HPGENSELECT also supports other methods for variable selection such as forward, backward, and stepwise selection methods. The STOP=SBC and CHOOSE=SBC functions specify the Schwarz Bayesian criterion to end the process of selection and to select variables. If the METHOD=LASSO is specified, but neither the CHOOSE= nor the STOP= option is specified, then the model in the last LASSO step is chosen as the final model. The Test partition is also not available for the LASSO method. The DETAILS=ALL statement requests that all information that is related to model selection be produced. Using minimum SBC criterion (3687.366), the resulting final model had only two elements: Intercept, and LowBirthWgt. None of the interactions are significant. In this case, the model in the last step had the smallest SBC statistic, therefore it was selected.

Table 9.6. Fit statistics for infant mortality selected model in 2003

Fit Statistics	Training	Validation
2 Log Likelihood	3654.11	1710.54
AIC (smaller is better)	3660.11	1720.54
AICC (smaller is better)	3660.11	1720.54
BIC (smaller is better)	3687.37	1761.74
Pearson Chi-Square	50587	29213
Pearson Chi-Square/DF	0.7747	1.0496
Average Square Error	0.005372	0.005695

Table 9.6 presents the Fit Statistics information for the selected model. Compared to Table 9.5, all statistics of the selected model show better performance. Thus, the selected model can better fit the infant mortality data.

Table 9.7 displays parameter estimates and standard errors of the model effects for the final model.

Table 9.7. Parameter estimates for infant mortality final model in 2003

Parameter	DF	Estimate
Intercept	1	-4.580326
LowBirthWgt No	1	-1.417116
LowBirthWgt Yes	1	1.420583

Using the OUTPUT statement in Program 9.2, you can store the linear predictors and the predicted probabilities resulted from the final model in a separate data set (Out). Since this data set also contains the ID variable that you added earlier to the data set in the first section of Program 9.1, therefore you can merge it to the covariates using the first section of Program 9.3 to obtain probability for any specific observation. For example, the probability of infant death for a person with the characteristics of Lowbirthwgt="Yes", Married="No", Agegroup=1, Race="Black", Drinking="Yes", Smoking="Yes", and Somecollege="No" in the model (second section of Program 9.3) is: 0.041.

Program 9.3: Merging Birthwgt and Out Data Sets for Estimationof Probability of a Specific Observation

```
/*Section 1*/
data out;
merge out birthwgt;
by id;
run;

/*Section 2*/
proc print data=out;
where lowbirthwgt="Yes" & married="No" & agegroup=1 &
race="Black" &
drinking="Yes" & smoking="Yes" & somecollege="No" ;
run;
```

Although LASSO is a superior method for variable selection compared to other methods, like other automatic selection methods, the context of a statistical problem or research is not considered as a factor, so the result of variable selection should cautiously be accepted (Efron et al., 2004).

References

Efron B., Hastie T., Tibshirani, R. 2004. Least angle regression, *Annals of Statistics* 32, 407–499.
SAS Institute Inc. 2015. SAS/STAT® 14.1 *User's Guide.* Cary, NC: SAS Institute Inc.
Schwarz G. 1978. Estimating the dimension of a model. *Annals of Statistics.* 6 (2): 461–464.
Steyerberg E. W. 2009. *Clinical Prediction Models.* Springer Science + Business Media, LLC. https://doi.org/10.1007/978-0-387-77244-8_2.
Tibshirani R. 1996. Regression Shrinkage and Selection via the lasso. *Journal of the Royal Statistical Society.* Series B (methodological). 58: 267–88.

Chapter 10

Machine Learning for Medical Diagnoses

Abstract

The analysis of clinical data allows us to comprehend the biological mechanisms that cause diseases and how risk factors impact their development. With a large amount of available data such as medical symptoms from various types of biochemical assays and imaging devices, clinicians can leverage machine learning (ML) algorithms to discover which features (variables) are more associated with the risk of appearance of a disease. Other reported applications of ML in healthcare are drug development and image analysis (Sordo, 2002), clinical diagnosis especially for rare disease (Ehsani-Moghaddam et al. 2018), prediction of diseases such as cancer (Shahid and Berta, 2019), interpretation of electrocardiograms (Bartosch-Harlid et al., 2008), and prediction of length of stay in hospital (Tsai et al., 2016). Machine learning algorithms are divided into several subcategories including supervised, unsupervised, and semi-supervised learning, transduction, reinforcement learning, and developmental learning, of which supervised and unsupervised learning techniques are the most widely applied algorithms in medical sciences.

In this chapter you will be introduced to several popular supervised learning algorithms. You will also compare different ML models for classification of breast cancer. Breast cancer is one of the most common cancers and is the second most widespread cancer after skin cancer diagnosed in women in the United States.

In recent years, survival rates have increased for this type of cancer, and the number of deaths associated with this disease is progressively declining, mainly because of factors such as earlier diagnosis, new treatment methods, and a better understanding of the nature of the disease. Therefore, any technique that supports health practitioners in clinical assessment and making a diagnosis as early as possible has the potential to make a significant positive impact on the cancer patient's life.

10.1. Objectives

The objectives of this chapter are: (1) to generate and evaluate an effective and accurate machine learning algorithm that uses minimum information from the breast cancer data to classify patients for malignant or benign cancer; (2) to assess and compare the relative efficiency of different machine learning models; and (3) to detect the features that are the most helpful in predicting malignant cancer.

10.2. Methodology

The focus of this chapter is on supervised machine learning algorithms. Supervised learning consists of prediction and classification algorithms. In general, supervised learning algorithms are trained on training data and after learning the patterns by preprocessing examples they are validated on validation (and sometimes on the test) data, then they predict/classify on target data. For this chapter, you will create several supervised learning models including a decision tree (DT) (Mohan, 2013), a Bayesian network augmented Naïve Bayes classifier (BAN) (Ehsani-Moghaddam et al., 2018), a support vector machine (SVM) (Rätsch et al., 2006), an artificial neural network (ANN) (Schmidhuber, 2015), and a logistic regression (LR) model and compare the performance of these algorithms for cancer type classification. Figure 10.1 is a flowchart that illustrates the main steps toward creation and validation of the final selected algorithm. The flowchart starts with making a data set and ends with the estimation of precision metrics for the ML algorithm that was selected. During construction of ML models, you may want to change the order of steps depending on different circumstances. For example, variable selection can be carried out before and/or after model comparison.

Using SAS studio version 3.8 or later that has access to a CAS library, SAS Enterprise Miner, and SAS Viya®, you can perform all tasks related to this chapter with no need for additional programming. Here SAS Enterprise Miner is used for the entire analysis. SAS Enterprise Miner has extensive capabilities for many aspects of data mining including text mining and machine learning process. It offers many ML-related tools including data partitioning, model assessment, feature selection, supervised learning models such as high-performance Bayesian networks, neural networks, random forests, and support vector machines, and unsupervised models such hieratical clustering, Principal Component Analysis, and text mining. Enterprise Miner is a process-flow-based and drag-and-drop task-oriented software that makes it easy to assemble many machine learning models or data mining procedures. For more information about the software refer to the SAS® Enterprise Miner user's guide in the References section.

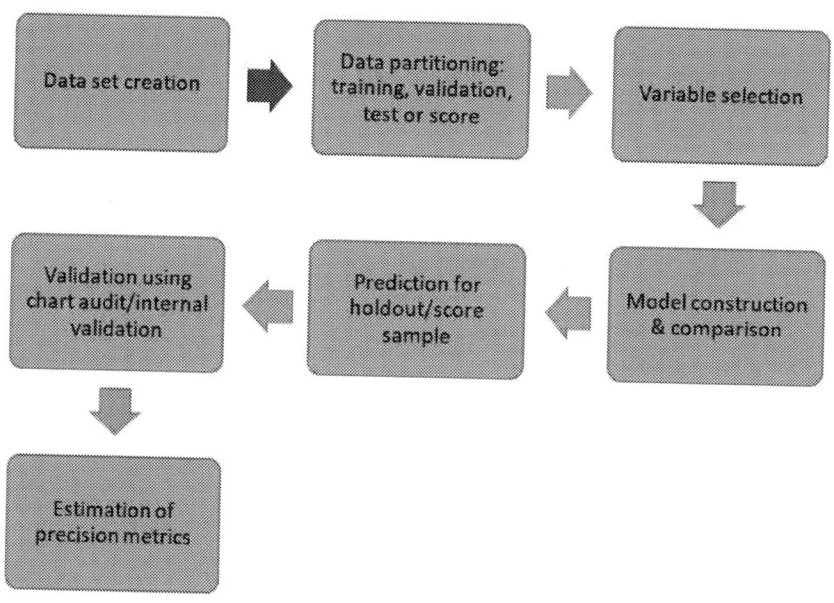

Figure 10.1. Flowchart of machine learning application for breast cancer classification.

10.2.1. Data Set

The data set (n=569) for this chapter is the Breast Cancer data set, which was created by Dr. Wolberg and his colleagues (1994). The data set and the characteristics of the features are publicly available from the UCI Machine Learning Repository[1].

According to this web site, features for the data set were computed from a digitized image of a fine needle aspirate of a breast mass. The mean and standard error were computed for each image, resulting in 30 features including the "worst" or largest (mean of the three largest values) variable.

---

[1] http://archive.ics.uci.edu/ml/datasets/breast+cancer+wisconsin+%28diagnostic%29.

For instance, field 3 is Mean Radius, field 13 is Radius SE, field 23 is Worst Radius. They describe characteristics of the cell nuclei present in the image. Other characteristics of the data set are:

- Number of instances: 569
- Number of attributes: 32 including id, diagnosis as dependent variable (m = malignant, b = benign), and 30 real-valued input features

Ten real-valued features are computed for each cell nucleus, including:

1. Radius (mean of distances from center to points on the perimeter)
2. Texture (standard deviation of gray-scale values)
3. Perimeter
4. Area
5. Smoothness (local variation in radius lengths)
6. Compactness (perimeter^2 / area -1.0)
7. Concavity (severity of concave portions of the contour)
8. Concave points (number of concave portions of the contour)
9. Symmetry
10. Fractal dimension (coastline approximation -1).

Prior to start working with this data, you should rename the following variables to the names that are acceptable for SAS:

- "concave points_mean" to "CP_mean"
- "concave points_se " to "CP_se"
- "concave points_worst" to "CP_worst"
- "fractal_dimension_mean" to "FD_mean"
- "fractal_dimension_se" to "FD_se"
- "fractal_dimension_worst" to "FD_worst"

10.2.2. Creating Project, Library, and Data Source

10.2.2.1. Creating Project and Diagram

After downloading the CSV file, you need to create a project and diagram first, because in SAS Enterprise Miner, all works are stored in projects and each project can contain several flow diagrams and information similar to the workflow in Figure 10.1. To create the project and diagram, follow these steps:

1. Launch SAS Enterprise Miner.
2. In the **Welcome to Enterprise Miner** window, click **New Project**.
3. When the **Create New Project Wizard** opens, choose the logical workspace server to use (e.g., SASApp) and click **Next**.
4. Enter **Breast Cancer** (or any name) as the **Project Name**. Then choose a SAS server directory for the project. The directory will be used to store all relevant data and information about your current project. Then click **Next**.
5. Review the summary information about the project and click **Finish**.

Next create a diagram by clicking on **Diagram** icon.

To access the data sets by SAS Enterprise Miner, you must also create a SAS library. Creating a new SAS library for SAS Enterprise Miner is easy and can be done by following steps:

1. Create a new folder where your Breast Cancer data set will be stored and enter a name for that. For this chapter name the library as ML. Then open the library wizard by clicking on the **File** menu and selecting **New** then **Library**.
2. Proceed through the steps in the Library Wizard. If you need to be granted directory access or if you are unsure about the details of your site configuration, contact your system administrator. At this step, the **Create New Library** option is automatically selected. Then click **Next**.
3. Enter the path to the directory where your Breast Cancer data set is stored then click **Finish**.

To utilize the CSV Breast Cancer data set, use the **File Import** node, which is located on the **Sample** tab on the Toolbar. Drag the File Import node on the diagram. You can import Microsoft Excel, SAS JMP, SPSS, Stata, CSV and Tab-Delimited and dBASE files using the File Import node. Click the ellipsis button for **Import File** and open the **File Import** window. Browse on the File Import window and navigate to the location of Breast Cancer file and click **Open** button on the Open window and then click **OK** on the File Import window. Run the File Import node.

10.2.2.2. Saving the Created SAS Table

The Save Data node which is located on the Utility tab can be used to save the SAS table that you created from CSV file into the ML library. This node enables you to save, for example the training, validation, test, score, or transaction data from any node to either a defined SAS library or a specified file path. Drag the **Save Data** node to the diagram and connect the File Import node to it by connecting the two nodes and placing the mouse pointer over the right side of the data source node until the indicator becomes a pencil. Then drag the pencil to the left edge of the StatExplore node. Then, release the mouse button as shown in Figure 10.2. Click the ellipsis button for **SAS Library Name** and choose the **ML library** (the library that you created for this project) and then run the node. This will save your SAS table into the ML library. After running any node, if it is outlined in a check mark inside a green circle that means that the process was successful, otherwise a red color denotes an error during the processing.

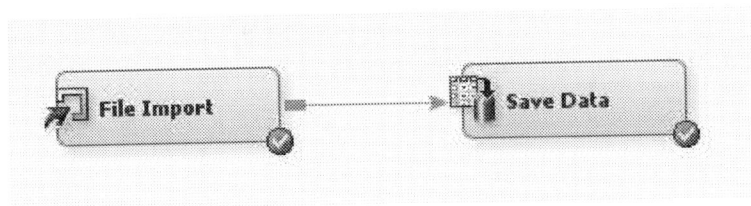

Figure 10.2. Connecting the file import node to the save data node.

10.2.2.3. Data Source

After importing the data, you must create a new Data Source using the Data Source Wizard by following these steps:

1. Click on the **File menu >> New >> Data Source**. You can also Right-click on the **Data Source** icon.
2. Proceed through the steps in the wizard. A SAS Table is automatically selected as the Source. Click **Next**. If you cannot see the Breast Cancer data set that you imported and saved, use **Browse table** to locate the data set in the ML library. Click Next. A Table Properties containing some basic information about the process of creating data source will be appeared. Click **Next**.
3. Select the **Advanced** option button and then click **Next**. Changing a feature role can be done by clicking on the value of that feature and selecting from the drop-down menu that appears. Change the value

of **Role** for the variables to match these descriptions: change **ID variable** role to **ID**, **Diagnosis** to **Target** and its **Level** to **Binary**, and all other variables should have Input role. Then click **Next**.
4. Select the **No** option button to indicate that you do not want to create models based on the values of decisions.
5. The role of the data source is automatically selected as **Raw**. Change the data source name to **Breast_Cancer** and click **Next** and then click **Finish**.

10.2.3. Creating a Flow Diagram

A flow diagram in Enterprise Miner can be created by adding nodes. To create a flow diagram for this project, follow these steps:

1. Click on **File Menu>>New>>Diagram**.
2. Enter a name for the diagram (e.g., Breast_Cancer) and click **OK**.
3. Create an input data node by dragging the Breast_Cancer data set into the workspace.

10.2.4. Data Exploration

Data exploration and descriptive statistics including summary statistics, and scatter plots for different features can easily be obtained using StatExplore node.

1. Select the **Explore** tab on the Toolbar and select the **StatExplore** node icon then drag the node into the workspace.
2. Connect the Breast_Cancer node to the StatExplore node. Select the StatExplore node. In the Properties Panel of the node, you can change statistics properties group. Right-click the **StatExplore** node and select **Run** and click **Yes** in the Confirmation window. After completing the processing, click **Results** on the window that appears and verify the results.

To save data for further analysis at this step or in any other step, use the Save Data node as described in Section 10.2.2.2. Drag the Save Data node from the Utility tab to the workspace and connect the StatExplore node to the

Save Data node. Then change the following properties of the Save Data node:

1. In the **Filename Prefix** property, enter **SavedData**.
2. Click the ellipsis button in the **SAS Library Name** property to open the **Select a SAS Library** window. Select **ML** and click OK.
3. Right-click the **Save Data** node and click **Run**.

10.2.5. Imputation and Transformation

The next steps are data imputation and data transformation, which can be carried out by the Impute and Transform Variables nodes, respectively. In SAS Enterprise Miner, models such as neural networks the entire observations that contain missing values will be dropped from analysis. This can reduce the size of your data set. To overcome this problem, you can impute missing values before fitting models. Since the Breast Cancer data set does not have any missing data, it does not need to do imputation. But in general, if you need to impute data for those data sets that contain missing observations, you can do so by following these steps:

1. Select the **Modify** tab on the Toolbar, select the **Impute** node and drag the node into the Diagram Workspace.
2. Connect the Save Data node to the Impute node.
3. In the **Properties** Panel of the node, scroll down to view the Train properties. For all interval variables, choose the value of **Default Input Method** and select **Median** from the drop-down menu. The values of missing interval variables (if any) are replaced by the median of the non-missing values, which are less sensitive to extreme values than the mean values.

Variable transformations can be used to stabilize variance, remove nonlinearity, and normalize data. For many models, transformations of the data can have an advantage of a better model fit. To transform variables, you can follow these steps:

1. From the **Modify** tab on the Toolbar, select the **Transform Variables** node icon and drag it into the **Workspace**.
2. Connect the Save Data node to the Transform Variables node.

Machine Learning for Medical Diagnoses

3. In the Properties Panel of the node click on the ellipses that represent the variables table. Select any row in the variable table that have the role Input and click on **Explore** tab to display the histogram of the variable in the panel. If variables have skewed distributions, they need to be transformed.
4. You can use log transformation or any other method to control skewness. For this example, use log transformation for the following features:
5. area_mean, compactness_mean, concavity_mean, CP_mean, radius_se, texture_se, perimeter_se, area_se, smoothness_se, compactness_se, concavity_se, symmetry_se, FD_se, texture_worst, area_worst, compactness_worst, concavity_worst, then click OK.
6. Run the Transform Variables node.

10.2.6. Variable Selection

To avoid overfitting the models, feature selection and removing unnecessary variables should be carried out before classification or prediction by model. Variable selection also reduces the number of input variables and saves computer resources, especially when there are too many variables. This can be done by different methods such as by Chi-square statistics of independent analysis and by variable importance (worth) based on computed importance values from Tree-based analysis as a surrogate model and then using positive predictive values of each feature. Chi-square statistics for interval variables can be carried out by binding the variables. To carry out variable selection in Enterprise Miner, use the Variable Selection node and follow these steps:

1. Select the Explore or HPDM tabs on the toolbar and drag the Variable Selection node icon into the Workspace.
2. Connect the Transform Variables node to the Variable Selection node.
3. Configure the Variable Selection Node by clicking and selecting the **Variable Selection** node in the workspace and then by going to the Properties Panel for the node and making the **Target Model** property to **Chi Square.**
4. Right-click the **Variable Selection** node, and press **Run**.

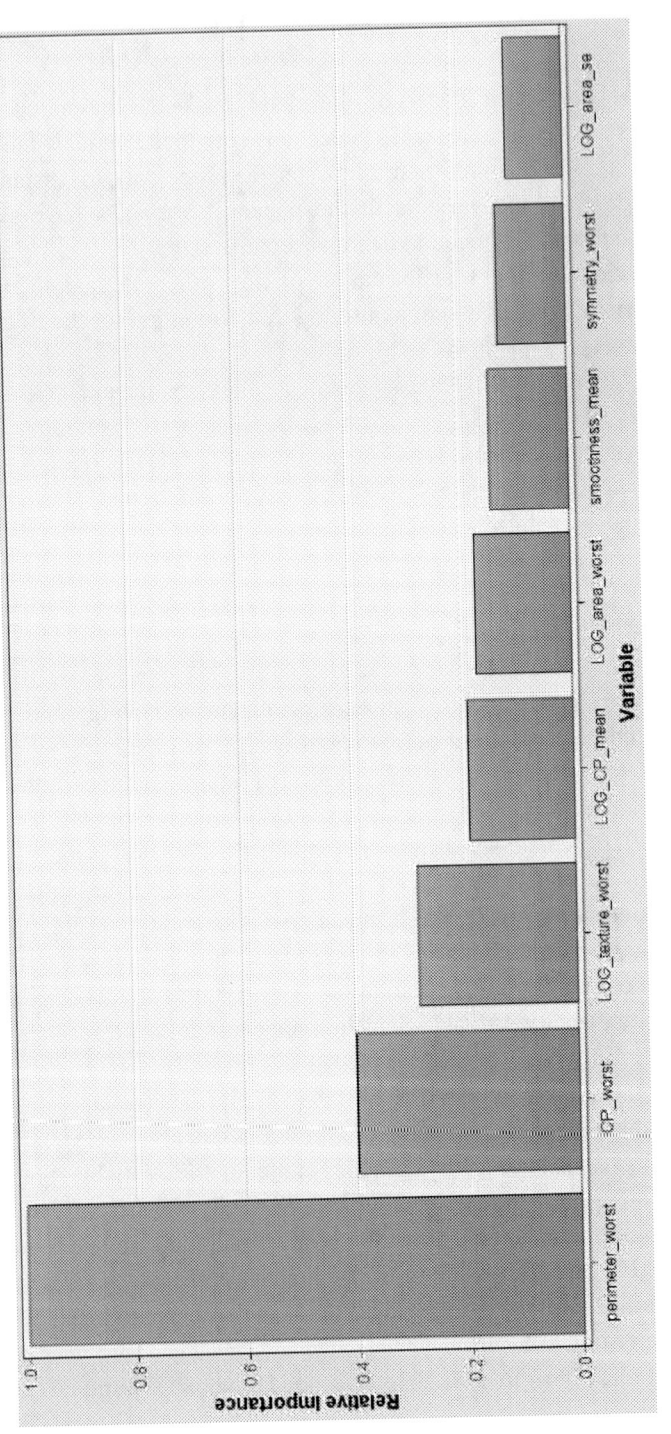

Figure 10.3. Variable importance plot for breast cancer data set.

Machine Learning for Medical Diagnoses 151

5. When processing completes, click Results and assess the Variable Selection table to see which features were selected. The status of variables in the Role column for variables that were not selected is changed from the Input to Rejected.

In this example, all features are rejected except CP_worst, Log_CP_mean, Log_area_se, Log_area_worst, Log_texture_worst, perimeter_worst, smoothness_mean, and symmetry_worst. Figure 10.3 displays the histogram of Variable Importance based on input features, scaled by their relative importance as predictors for the diagnosis target variable.

10.2.7. Multicollinearity

In any machine learning algorithm, we assume conditional independence among features. In order to test this assumption and remove highly correlated features that may cause multicollinearity problems, you can estimate the degree of relationship among features. The results of this part of study can be summarized into a correlation matrix heatmap. If the coefficient correlation analysis using all features in the data set does not show any substantial correlation among features, indicating that there is no multicollinearity among predictors in the data set and that the assumption of independency among attributes is valid, otherwise the correlated features need to be identified and fixed.

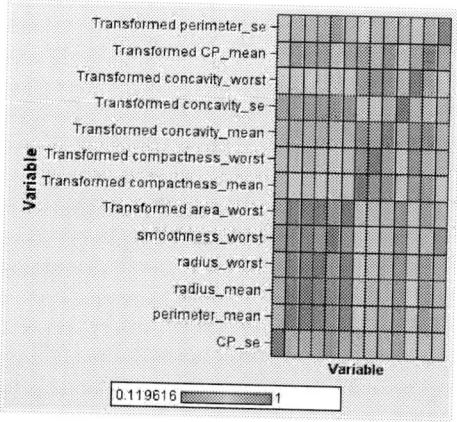

Figure 10.4. Heatmap and the degree of correlation between variables in breast cancer data set.

A correlation matrix heatmap can be obtained using the Variable Clustering node. Connect the Variable Selection node from the previous section to the Variable Clustering node and then run the node. After the results are ready, click **View >> Model >> Variable Correlation**. In a heatmap, the degree of correlation between variables is illustrated by the intensity of red color (Figure 10.4). Those variables with minimum correlation are shown with blue color. For the purpose of this training, all variables are selected regardless of their correlation results.

10.2.8. Data Partitioning

You can use the Validation Set Approach technique to assess the efficacy of the designed algorithm or to compare the performance of the created ML models. In this approach you randomly partition 40% of the dataset as the training set, 30% as the validation set and 30% as the test set. This partitioning ratio is arbitrary and can be changed to, for example, 70% as training and 30% as validation and without testing if the data set is not large enough. The training set is used to create the model. The performance of the model is validated and confirmed by the validation set, and the prediction will be carried out on the test data set. When the data set is big enough, a portion of data should be held aside as the holdout sample for the subsequent validation of the outcomes and final performance assessment. A key issue with practical application of machine learning in healthcare is the lack of enough data to support training, validation, and the final test. The validation, test, and holdout samples should not be used in any learning process or creation of ML algorithm. At the end of this chapter and after you selected the best model, you use Score_Data, which has been provided for scoring practices to predict scores for tumor type and then you compare the scores from the model with those from the gold standard observations using a 2 X 2 confusion matrix.

To partition data using SAS Enterprise Miner, follow these steps:

1. Select the **Sample** or **HPDM** tabs on the Toolbar.
2. Select the **Data Partition** node icon and drag it into the workspace.
3. Connect the Variable Selection node to the Data Partition node.
4. In the Properties Panel of Data Partition node, click on the value of **Training, Validation,** and **Test**, and enter **40.0, 30.0** and **30.0,**

respectively. This proportion is also default ratio from the Enterprise Miner.
5. Right-click on the **Data Partition** node and then run the program.

For the reproducibility and consistency of the results from this part of program, you can assign a random number (any number) in the Random Seed section of the Properties Panel of Data Partition node so that in future you can get the same random partitioned data sets. Remember to check the LOG tab for any possible errors.

10.2.9. Building and Assessing Models

You will apply the training data set and its features to compute the conditional posterior probabilities for the diagnosis categorical dependent variable for all patients in the BC data set. You will construct several different learning models: a linear regression (LR), a decision tree (DT), a Bayesian Network Augmented Naïve Bayes Classifier (BAN), a support vector machine (SVM), and an artificial neural network (ANN) in the high-performance (HP) environment. You will also compare the performance of these algorithms for breast cancer classification.

To construct these models, from the HPDM tab on the Toolbar, select the icon nodes of these models and drag them into the Diagram Workspace. Then connect the Data Partition node to the nodes of all these models. Next, in the Properties Panel of these model nodes apply the following changes:

- For LR, use the stepwise selection method for model selection with logit link function for training the model. The selection criterion to determine the order in which effects entered or left at each step of the selection will be significant level of the effects.
- For the DT model, entropy is the splitting criterion to regulate the best splits on inputs given the Diagnosis target, with 100 interval bins and the number of subsets that a splitting rule could produce is set to two with maximum depth of 10 and leaf size of eight. The subtrees creation and pruning are carried out using cost-complexity (the subtree with a minimum leaf-penalized average square error).
- For the BAN algorithm, variables should be prescreened and selected using Chi-square independence test for input variables and by P-vale=0.5 as significant level.

- For the SVM, the interior point is as optimization technique with a linear kernel during training.
- For the ANN model, enable direct connections from the input units to the output units by using one layer with direct architecture, with three hidden neurons and with identity activation functions for the ANN algorithm, which results in minimum validation average squared error and minimum sum of squared error compared with other architectures.

10.2.10. Model Comparison

The performances of these models are compared by the Validation Set Approach technique, which is carried out by partitioning randomly the data set as training, validation, and test set as discussed in Section 10.2.9. As mentioned earlier, for this project the Score_Data set serves you as a hold-out sample for prediction.

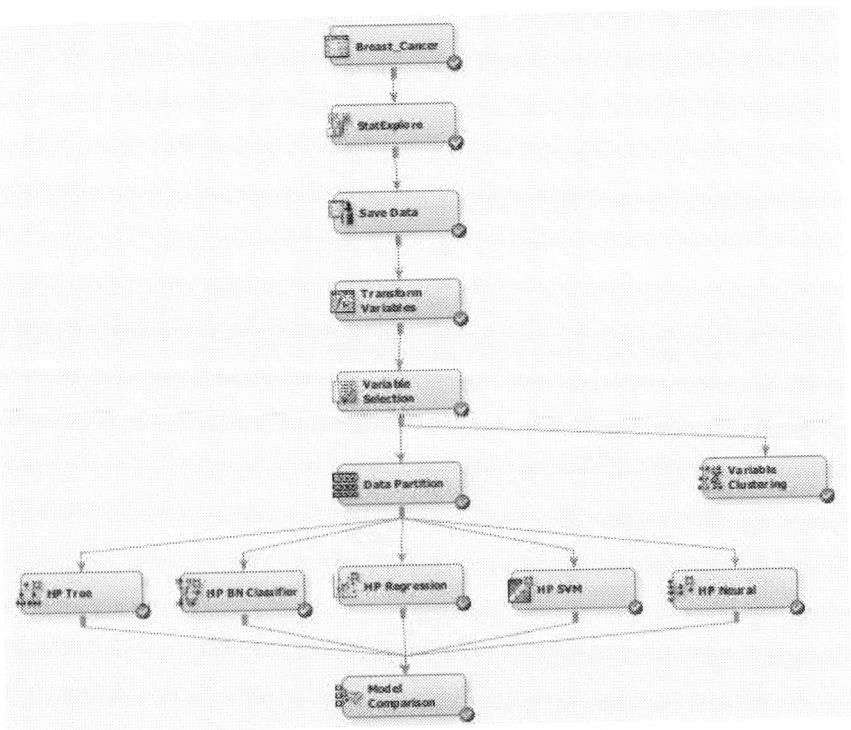

Figure 10.5. Model comparison for breast cancer classification.

For model comparison, several accuracy parameters such as average squared error, misclassification rate, average, and sum of squared error of models, receiver operating characteristic curve (ROC) index, Gini coefficient and information gain (the knowledge gained by the algorithm to solve classification problem) are used for performance comparison. A Gini coefficient is a measure of the uniformity of a distribution. In the perspective of modeling, the Gini coefficient is used to compare the event rates across the attributes. The model with the highest ROC index, Gini coefficient, Gain value, true positive, true negative, and the lowest error parameters, misclassification, false positive, and false negative is selected as the champion model for estimating dependent variable status. To be able to do model comparison, you need to use the Model Comparison node. Drag a Model Comparison node from the Assess tab to the workspace and connect each modeling node to the Model Comparison node and right-click on the **Model Comparison** node and select **Run** (Figure 10.5).

The Output window in the Model Comparison Results reveals the assessment statistics for all models. According to this output, the ANN model (Figure 10.6) has been selected as the best model based on the validation misclassification rate and other parameters.

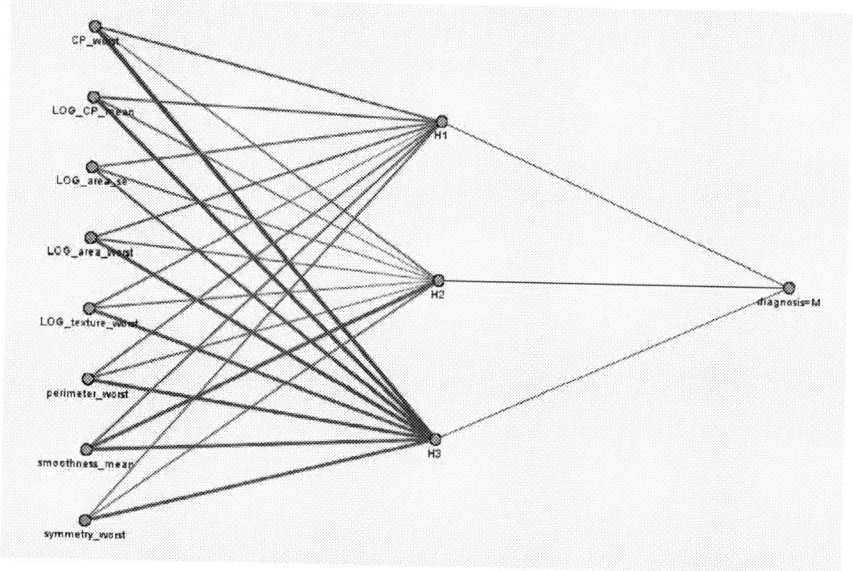

Figure 10.6. Final architecture of artificial neural networks with one-layer, direct edges and three hidden neurons of the breast cancer data. Features are input and the diagnosis type of tumor is output.

An ANN model is a nonlinear learning and information processing system inspired by the natural and biological function of the human brain to perform specific tasks such as classification, clustering, and speech and pattern recognition. The main characteristics of ANNs are their ability to learn complex nonlinear input-output relationships, use sequential training procedures, and adapt themselves to the data with potential advantage of using hidden layers for automatic feature combinations, which can capture complex information.

A standard neural network consists of many simple, connected processors called units, each producing a sequence of real-valued activations and arranged in a series of layers (Figure 10.6).

The supervised ANN learning utilizes a set of data pairs (x: input variable, y: output variable) where x∈X and y∈Y to create a function of f: X→Y in the acceptable class of functions that matches the examples. The basic neural network model, which can be described as a series of functional transformations can be written as:

$$a_j = \sum_{i=1}^{D} w_{ji}^{(1)} x_i + w_{j0}^{(1)} \qquad (1)$$

where j = 1, ..., M. The superscript (1) indicates that the corresponding parameters are in the first layer of the network, parameter $w_{ji}^{(1)}$ is weight and $w_{j0}^{(1)}$ is bias. The parameters a_j will be transformed using a differentiable, nonlinear activation function h (·) (sigmoidal functions such as the logistic sigmoid or tanh function) to produce:

$$z_j = h(a_j) \qquad (2)$$

In the context of neural networks, z_j again linearly combined to give output unit activations:

$$a_k = \sum_{j=1}^{M} w_{kj}^{(2)} z_j + w_{k0}^{(2)} \qquad (3)$$

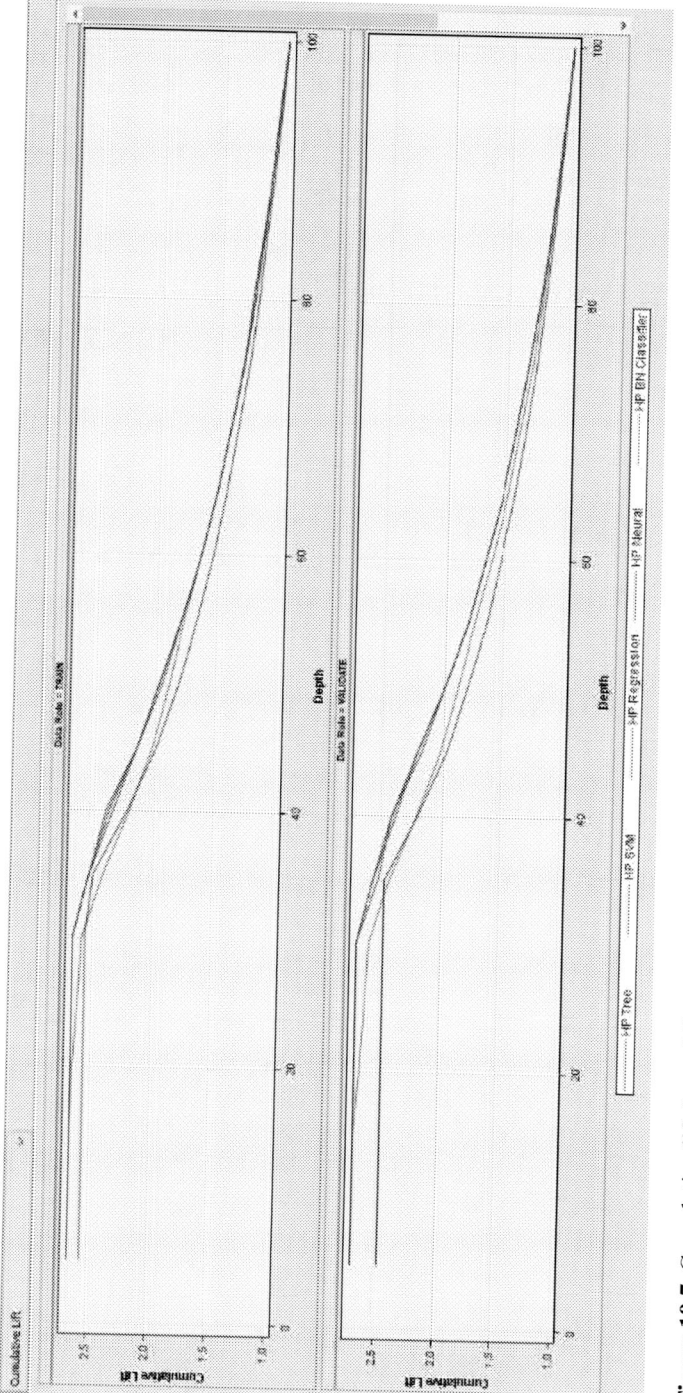

Figure 10.7. Cumulative lift from different models in breast cancer data set.

where k = 1, ..., K and K is the total number of outputs. This transformation corresponds to the second layer of the network, and $w_{k0}^{(2)}$ are also bias parameters. Eventually, the output unit activations are transformed using an appropriate activation function to give a set of network outputs y_k (Bishop, 2006).

Layers in ANN can be divided into an input layer, which covers the units that accept input from the outside by learning process; output layer, which covers units that return to the information about learning tasks; hidden layer, which are the units located between input and output layers and they convert the input information into output using appropriate mathematical procedures by linear relationship or often in a non-linear way.

In the Model Comparison node, click on **Results** and select **Cumulative Lift** from the drop-down menu of Score Ranking plots. The ANN model has relatively higher lift values than other models for both Training and Validation data sets (Figure 10.7).

10.2.11. Scoring a Data Set Using the Selected Model

Since the overall performance of the ANN model was superior to all other models, thus, you can use the scoring code from this model to classify or predict the target values for a new data set.

For this training, use the Score_Data that is provided for diagnosis classification.

Import the Score_Data as outlined in Section 10.2.2.2 and add a Score node from the Assess tab to the Diagram Workspace and connect the Save Data node, which contains Score_Data to the Score node.

Next, connect the Model Comparison node to the Score node and run the node. At this point, your process flow should look like Figure 10.8.

In the Score node result, you can see the scoring code. The predicted or classified scores for the diagnosis dependent variable from this section will automatically be saved in a folder.

To see the location of saved scores or to see the predicted values, you can click on the Exported Data icon of the Property panel of Score node.

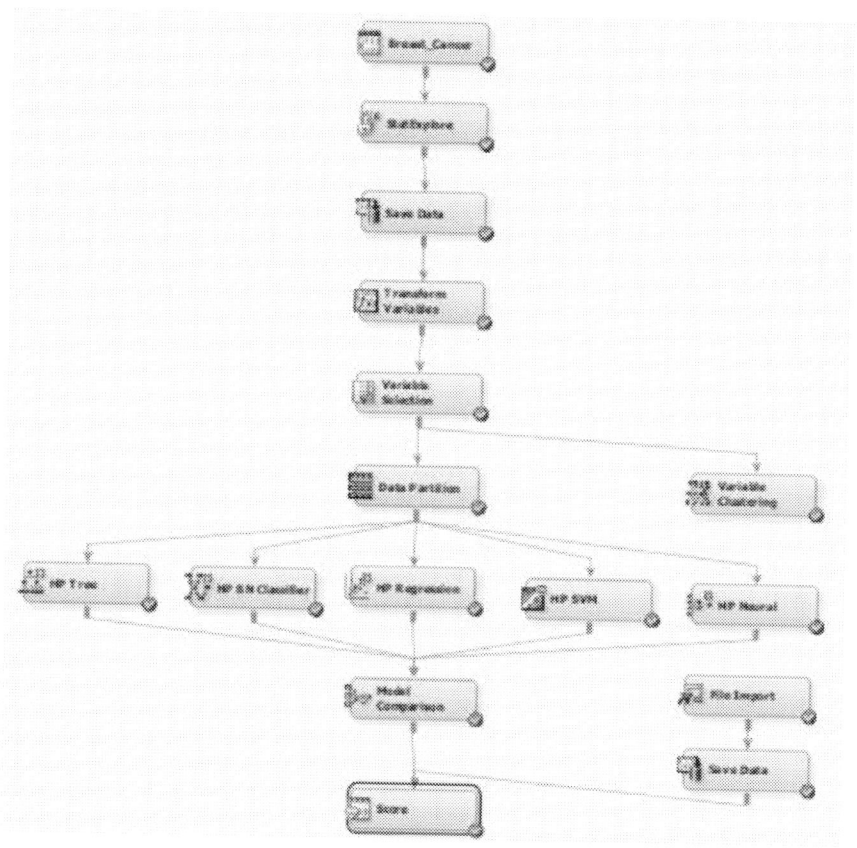

Figure 10.8. Scoring a new data set for breast cancer classification.

10.2.12. Estimation of Precision Metrics

Suppose you need to validate the final classification results and compare the classified cases that you obtained from the ANN model for the Score_Data with the results from a gold standard data such as the chart audit data set from patients. Suppose also after comparison; you found out that out of 100 patients in Score_Data, the ANN model classified 62 patients with malignant and 38 patients with benign cancer, which compared to the gold standard results the ANN model classified three cases as false negative and two cases as false positive. To estimate precision metrics for ANN model and calculate accuracy statistics such as sensitivity, specificity and so on, Program 10.1

can be used. In this program M (malignant) and B (benign) cases have been replaced with 1 and 0, respectively.

Program 10.1: Estimation of Precision Metrics for ANN Model

```
data validation;
      input ANN$  Chart$  count;
      datalines;
      0  0   35
      0  1    3
      1  0    2
      1  1   60
      ;
      proc sort data=validation;
      by descending ANN descending Chart Count;
      run;
      proc freq data=validation order=data;
      weight count;
      tables ANN*Chart/nopercent norow nocol nocum;;
      run;

         title 'Sensitivity';
      proc freq data=validation;
         where Chart="1";
         weight count;
         tables ANN / binomial(level="1");
         exact binomial;
         run;

      title 'Specificity';
      proc freq data=validation;
         where Chart="0";
         weight count;
         tables ANN / binomial(level="0");
         exact binomial;
         run;

      title 'Positive predictive value';
      proc freq data=validation;
         where ANN="1";
         weight count;
         tables Chart / binomial(level="1");
         exact binomial;
         run;

      title 'Negative predictive value';
      proc freq data=validation;
```

```
        where ANN="0";
        weight count;
        tables Chart / binomial(level="0");
        exact binomial;
        run;

     title 'Accuracy';
data acc;
        set validation;
        if (ANN and Chart) or
           (not ANN and not Chart) then acc="1";
        else acc="0";
        run;
    proc freq;
        weight count;
        tables acc / binomial(level="1");
        exact binomial;
        run;

ods graphics on;
        title 'Kappa';
         proc freq data=validation order=data;
        tables ANN*Chart  / norow nocol nopercent
  agree ;
        test kappa;
           weight count;
        run;
                1. ods graphics off;
```

The results of cross-validation of the score dataset by comparison of ANN classified cases and cases classified by the gold standard system are expressed by accuracy and other relevant statistics that are calculated from a confusion matrix for binary classifiers:

$$\text{Accuracy} = \frac{TP+TN}{TP+TN+FP+FN} \tag{4}$$

$$\text{Sensitivity} = \frac{TP}{TP+FN} \tag{5}$$

$$\text{Specificity} = \frac{TN}{TN+FP} \tag{6}$$

$$\text{PPV} = \frac{TP}{TP+FP} \tag{7}$$

$$\text{NPV} = \frac{\text{TN}}{\text{TN} + \text{FN}} \qquad (8)$$

where TP, TN, FP, FN, PPV and NPV are true positive, true negative, false positive, false negative, positive predictive value, and negative predictive value, respectively. Table 10.1 reports the results of performance evaluation of the ANN model in a 2 × 2 contingency table by comparison between predicted values from the ANN algorithm and observed values from a fictional chart audit as gold standard. According to Table 10.1, there were 95 (95.0%) correct classifications (35 for "Benign" and 60 for "Malignant", along the diagonal) and 5 (5.0%) incorrect classifications (2 for "Benign" and 3 for "Malignant", along the vertical). The overall accuracy, Kappa, sensitivity, specificity, positive predictive value, and negative predictive value of the ANN predictive model for the Cancer Data set are 0.95 (95% CI: 0.91, 0.99), 0.89 (95% CI: 0.80, 0.98), 0.95 (95% CI: 0.90, 1.0), 0.95 (95% CI: 0.87, 1.0), 0.97 (95% CI: 0.92, 1.0) and 0.92 (95% CI: 0.84, 1.0), respectively.

Table 10.1. ANN model performance

	Classified Observations from the Gold Standard System		
Predicted by ANN	B	M	Row total
B	35	3	38
M	2	60	62
Column total	37	63	100
Accuracy with 95% CI	0.95 (95% CI: 0.91, 0.99)		
Cohen's Kappa with 95% CI	0.89 (95% CI: 0.80, 0.98)		
Sensitivity with 95% CI	0.95 (95% CI: 0.90, 1.0)		
Specificity with 95% CI	0.95 (95% CI: 0.87, 1.0)		
PPV with 95% CI	0.97 (95% CI: 0.92, 1.0)		
NPV with 95% CI	0.92 (95% CI: 0.84, 1.0)		

PPV: Positive predictive value; NPV: Negative predictive value.

Conclusion

In the breast cancer data set of patients, the ANN algorithm and eight selected features from the data set, which applied to the diagnosis variable using SAS Enterprise Miner yields a better performance as compared to other classifiers. The ANN appears to be an efficient algorithm for classifying breast cancer cases. As EHR is becoming more common in healthcare systems, ANN and other machine learning models may provide an efficient way to better estimate the burden of different diseases and provided needed opportunities to address important existing care gaps.

References

Bartosch-Harlid A., Andersson B., Aho U., Nilsson J., Andersson R. Artificial neural networks in pancreatic disease. *Br J Surg.* 2008; 95(7):817–26.

Bishop C. *Pattern recognition and machine learning (Information Science and Statistics).* Springer-Verlag Berlin, Heidelberg. 2006, ISBN:0387310738.

Ehsani-Moghaddam B., Queenan J. A., MacKenzie J., Birtwhistle R. V. Mucopolysaccharidosis type II detection by Naïve Bayes Classifier: an example of patient classification for a rare disease using electronic medical records from the Canadian Primary Care Sentinel Surveillance Network. *PLOS ONE.* 2018; https://doi.org/10.1371/journal.pone.0209018.

Kalyan K., Jakhia B., Lele R. D., Joshi M. and Chowdhary A. Artificial Neural Network application in the diagnosis of disease conditions with liver ultrasound images. *Adv Bioinformatics.* 2014; https://doi.org/10.1155/2014/708279.

Mohan V. Decision Trees: *A comparison of various algorithms for building Decision Trees.* 2013; Available from: http://cs.jhu.edu/~vmohan3/document/ai_dt.pdf.

Rätsch G., Sonnenburg S. and Schäfer C. Learning Interpretable SVMs for Biological Sequence Classification. *BMC Bioinformatics.* 2006; 7(Suppl 1): S9. https://doi.org/10.1186/1471-2105-7-S1-S9.

SAS Institute Inc. 2017. *Getting Started with SAS® Enterprise Miner™ 14.3.* Cary, NC: SAS Institute Inc.

Schmidhuber, J. Deep Learning in Neural Networks: An Overview. *Neural Networks.* 2015; 61: 85–117. https://doi.org/10.1016/j.neunet.2014.09.003.

Shahid N., Rappon T., Berta W. Applications of artificial neural networks in health care organizational decision-making: A scoping review. *PLOS ONE.* 2019; https://doi.org/10.1371/journal.pone.0212356.

Sordo M. *Introduction to Neural Networks in Healthcare.* 2002; http://www.openclinical.org/docs/int/neuralnetworks011.pdf.

Tsai, P.-F. (Jennifer), Chen, P.-C., Chen, Y.-Y., Song, H.-Y., Lin, H.-M., Lin, F.-M., & Huang, Q.-P. Length of Hospital Stay Prediction at the Admission Stage for Cardiology Patients Using Artificial Neural Network. *J Healthc Eng.* 2016; https://doi.org/10.1155/2016/7035463.

Wolberg W. H., Street W. N., and Mangasarian O. L. Machine learning techniques to diagnose breast cancer from fine-needle aspirates. *Cancer Letters,* 1994, 77. 163-171.

Index

A

adverse effects, 70, 71, 72, 73, 77, 78, 79
adverse event, 79, 80, 83
age, ix, 12, 13, 14, 43, 49, 55, 56, 70, 74, 76, 79, 80, 81, 86, 87, 88, 89, 91, 92, 93, 94, 95, 96, 97, 98, 99, 100, 101, 104, 105, 106, 107, 112, 113, 114, 115, 116, 117, 118, 122
algorithm, 120, 121, 122, 124, 135, 142, 151, 152, 153, 154, 155, 162
allergy, 13, 60, 62, 64
arthralgia, 75, 76, 77, 78, 80
artificial neural network (ANN), 142, 153, 154, 155, 156, 158, 159, 160, 161, 162
assessment, 14, 126, 142, 152, 155
asthenia, 75, 77, 78, 80
asthma, 104, 106, 108, 109, 110
audit, 122, 124, 125, 159, 162
authentication, 15, 18, 21

B

Bayesian Network Augmented Naïve Bayes Classifier (BAN), 142, 153
benign, 142, 144, 159
bias, 8, 59, 136, 156, 158
body mass index (BMI), 12, 13, 51
bounds, 94, 95, 115
breast cancer, 141, 142, 143, 150, 151, 153, 154, 155, 157, 159, 162, 163

C

cancer, 141, 142, 143, 159, 163
Chronic Obstructive Pulmonary Disease (COPD), 49, 104, 105, 106, 107, 108, 109, 110, 111, 112, 113, 114, 115, 116, 117, 118, 119, 122, 123, 124, 125, 126, 127, 128
classes, 33, 88, 96, 101
classification, 79, 119, 120, 121, 122, 124, 125, 131, 141, 142, 143, 149, 153, 154, 155, 156, 158, 159, 163
clinical data, 141
computer, 16, 18, 134, 149
configuration, 19, 21, 145
cross-validation, 120, 122, 124, 126, 127, 128, 161
crude prevalence, 86, 89, 94, 95, 96, 104, 106, 107, 113, 115
Crude Prevalence Estimation, 86, 88, 105, 106

D

data set, ix, 6, 8, 9, 13, 15, 16, 21, 22, 23, 25, 27, 28, 29, 30, 31, 32, 33, 34, 35, 36, 37, 40, 43, 44, 45, 46, 47, 48, 49, 50, 51, 52, 54, 55, 56, 59, 61, 70, 71, 74, 77, 86, 89, 90, 91, 96, 103, 106, 108, 110, 112, 115, 119, 120, 122, 124, 126, 133, 134, 135, 136, 137, 138, 142, 143, 145, 146, 147, 148, 150, 151, 152, 153, 154, 157, 158, 159, 161, 162
database, vii, ix, 5, 7, 9, 12, 15, 16, 18, 20, 21, 22, 23, 24, 25, 27, 29, 43, 44, 45, 57, 58, 59, 70, 87, 115, 119, 129
decision support systems, 6, 119
decision tree (DT), 142, 153
dependent variable, 6, 7, 12, 131, 132, 144, 153, 155, 158
diseases, ix, 7, 13, 69, 85, 86, 103, 108, 119, 141, 163

Index

distribution, 34, 70, 77, 79, 87, 131, 132, 133, 155

E

Electronic Health Record (EHR), vii, ix, 1, 3, 4, 5, 6, 7, 8, 9, 10, 11, 12, 13, 14, 15, 18, 20, 21, 22, 23, 24, 25, 27, 28, 29, 35, 38, 43, 44, 45, 46, 48, 51, 54, 57, 58, 59, 61, 67, 85, 86, 89, 103, 119, 120, 124, 163
Electronic Medical Record (EMR), ix, 3
environment, 16, 24, 25, 31, 153
extraction, 9, 27, 69, 85

F

false negative, 119, 121, 125, 155, 159, 162
false positive, 119, 121, 125, 155, 159, 162
formula, 7, 93, 99, 122
FREQ, 31, 32, 53, 77, 79, 96, 124

G

gold standard, 119, 120, 122, 125, 126, 152, 159, 161, 162

H

health, ix, 3, 4, 6, 9, 10, 11, 14, 51, 70, 86, 89, 104, 107, 129, 131, 141, 163
health information, 4, 10, 11
Health Information Management Systems Society (HIMSS), 4, 14
healthcare, ix, 3, 4, 6, 9, 11, 14, 15, 24, 43, 44, 51, 57, 58, 59, 69, 70, 86, 87, 89, 104, 105, 107, 115, 118, 119, 120, 131, 141, 152, 163
height, 8, 12, 36, 37, 38, 119

I

icon, 29, 145, 146, 147, 148, 149, 152, 153, 158
identification, 4, 48, 51

independent variable, 7, 8, 12, 131, 133, 136
infant mortality, 133, 135, 136, 137, 138
International Classification of Disease (ICD) codes, ix, 44

L

learning, 120, 141, 142, 152, 153, 156, 158, 163
linear regression (LR), 142, 153

M

machine learning (ML), x, 8, 12, 131, 141, 142, 143, 145, 146, 148, 151, 152, 163
management, ix, 4, 11, 15, 51
matrix, 7, 120, 151, 152, 161
medical, ix, 3, 4, 6, 51, 61, 69, 101, 119, 141, 163
medication, ix, 12, 21, 22, 51, 60, 63, 64, 104, 108, 111
Microsoft, ix, 15, 40, 145
Microsoft SQL server, ix
models, x, 127, 131, 132, 134, 141, 142, 147, 148, 149, 152, 153, 154, 155, 157, 158, 163
Multiple Logistic Regression (MLR), 131, 132, 133

N

nausea, 75, 77, 78
neural network, 142, 148, 153, 155, 156, 163
nodes, 146, 147, 148, 153

P

pain, 69, 71, 72
partition, 134, 136, 137, 152
password, 18, 21, 24
physicians, 6, 8, 105
population, 8, 15, 85, 86, 87, 88, 89, 95, 96, 97, 99, 100, 101, 103, 104, 119
PRINT, 31, 32, 55

probability, 34, 122, 125, 131, 133, 134, 135, 138
programming, ix, 15, 22, 69, 80, 86, 88, 105, 106, 108, 119, 120, 142
project, 35, 51, 120, 144, 145, 146, 147, 154

R

race, 134, 137, 138
rash, 75, 76, 77, 78, 79, 80, 81, 82
reactions, 69, 70, 79
regression, x, 93, 131, 139, 142, 153
requirements, 6, 9, 10, 14
researchers, ix, 6, 8, 69, 119
resources, 6, 9, 83, 120, 126, 149
response, 12, 131, 132, 133, 135
risk, x, 9, 12, 69, 70, 79, 82, 87, 95, 101, 131, 136, 141
rule-based system, 86, 104, 120, 121, 125

S

SAS, vii, ix, 13, 15, 16, 20, 22, 23, 24, 25, 27, 28, 29, 30, 31, 34, 35, 36, 38, 39, 40, 41, 43, 44, 45, 49, 52, 54, 55, 56, 69, 70, 79, 83, 88, 93, 102, 127, 131, 132, 139, 142, 144, 145, 146, 148, 152, 162, 163, 173
SAS program, ix, 15, 27, 28, 35, 69
security, 3, 5, 10, 11, 14
sensitivity, x, 7, 70, 120, 121, 125, 127, 159, 162
sex, ix, 14, 33, 34, 35, 36, 37, 38, 70, 74, 76, 79, 80, 81, 82, 86, 87, 88, 89, 90, 92, 93, 94, 95, 96, 97, 99, 100, 101, 104, 106, 107, 112, 113, 114, 115, 116, 117, 118, 122, 127, 128
signs, 4, 94, 115
smoking, 12, 32, 37, 39, 40, 134, 137, 138
software, ix, 3, 15, 25, 54, 69, 88, 96, 97, 101, 143
SQL (Structured Query Language), 15, 16, 17, 18, 20, 21, 24, 25, 37, 44, 48, 64
standard deviation, 32, 34, 93, 127, 144
standard error, 32, 100, 136, 138, 143

standardization, x, 87, 88, 100
statistics, 32, 34, 85, 86, 89, 92, 93, 103, 113, 114, 120, 136, 137, 138, 147, 149, 155, 159, 161
storage, 15, 22, 25, 35
structure, 3, 5, 6, 13, 15
subset, 27, 31, 35, 36, 37, 38, 39, 47, 48, 55, 88, 89, 90, 106, 107, 108, 134, 135, 153
support vector machine (SVM), 142, 153, 154
surveillance, 9, 69, 102, 118, 119, 163
symptoms, 4, 12, 13, 71, 72, 119, 141

T

target, 71, 72, 142, 151, 153, 158
techniques, ix, 3, 10, 14, 44, 69, 72, 87, 120, 132, 141, 163
test data, 16, 134, 152
testing, 134, 135, 152
training, 134, 135, 142, 146, 152, 153, 154, 156, 158
transformation, 148, 149, 156, 158
Type I error, 120, 121, 127

U

United States, 58, 65, 95, 96, 101, 133, 141
UNIVARIATE, 34, 35

V

vaccine, 13, 22, 60, 63, 64, 70, 74, 78, 79, 80, 81, 83, 119
validation, x, 20, 119, 120, 122, 123, 124, 126, 127, 128, 134, 135, 142, 146, 152, 154, 155, 160, 161
variables, ix, 3, 7, 8, 12, 13, 28, 29, 30, 31, 32, 33, 34, 35, 36, 37, 39, 43, 45, 48, 49, 52, 56, 57, 61, 70, 71, 74, 79, 88, 91, 106, 108, 111, 112, 115, 131, 132, 133, 135, 136, 137, 141, 144, 147, 148, 149, 151, 152, 153

About the Author

Dr. Behrouz Ehsani-Moghaddam

Dr. Behrouz Ehsani-Moghaddam is a senior statistician at Abbott Point of Care and adjunct professor at Queen's University and has more than 16 years of experience working with SAS to solve the most important biostatistical challenges. He has more than 35 published papers in peered-reviewed journals. He lives in Ottawa, Canada, with his wife and family.